NATIONAL INSTITUTE SOCIAL
SERVICES LIBRARY

Volume 6

THE FIELD TRAINING OF
SOCIAL WORKERS

THE FIELD TRAINING OF SOCIAL WORKERS

A Survey

S. CLEMENT BROWN AND
E. R. GLOYNE

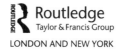

LONDON AND NEW YORK

First published in 1966 by George Allen & Unwin Ltd

This edition first published in 2022
by Routledge
4 Park Square, Milton Park, Abingdon, Oxon OX14 4RN
605 Third Avenue, New York, NY 10017

Routledge is an imprint of the Taylor & Francis Group, an informa business

© 1966 by Taylor & Francis.

British Library Cataloguing in Publication Data
A catalogue record for this book is available from the British Library

ISBN: 978-1-03-203381-5 (Set)
ISBN: 978-1-00-321681-0 (Set) (ebk)
ISBN: 978-1-03-204804-8 (Volume 6) (hbk)
ISBN: 978-1-03-204810-9 (Volume 6) (pbk)
ISBN: 978-1-00-319474-3 (Volume 6) (ebk)

DOI: 10.4324/9781003194743

Publisher's Note
The publisher has gone to great lengths to ensure the quality of this reprint but points out that some imperfections in the original copies may be apparent.

Disclaimer
The publisher has made every effort to trace copyright holders and would welcome correspondence from those they have been unable to trace.

THE FIELD TRAINING
OF SOCIAL WORKERS

A SURVEY

BY

S. CLEMENT BROWN

AND

E. R. GLOYNE

London

GEORGE ALLEN & UNWIN LTD

RUSKIN HOUSE · MUSEUM STREET

PRINTED IN GREAT BRITAIN

in 11 on 12 point Fournier type

BY C. TINLING AND CO. LTD

LIVERPOOL, LONDON AND PRESCOT

ACKNOWLEDGEMENTS

We are grateful to the members of the Advisory Committee both for their wise guidance in shaping this inquiry and also for our freedom to present findings for which only the authors are responsible.

Thought and time have been generously given by many busy people. To social workers, academic staff, members of professional organizations and students we offer our warm thanks for their interest and ready response. We also owe much to those who promote training for social work, particularly our colleagues at the National Institute for Social Work Training.

To Margery Seward we are greatly indebted for help in the analysis of records and the index, and to Margaret Johnson for the competence of her maps.

S.C.B.

E.R.G.

MEMBERS OF THE ADVISORY COMMITTEE

Mr R. Huws Jones: *Chairman*

Miss G. M. Aves, C.B.E.	Mr G. Newton
Miss Z. Butrym	Mrs K. Russell
Miss O. Chandler	Mr R. W. Speirs
Mr David Jones	Miss E. C. Warren
Miss K. M. Lewis	Mr. R. C. Wright

Dame Eileen Younghusband

FOREWORD

———

TRAINED social workers are in demand today as never before, to work with children in trouble, with old people and those who are handicapped in mind or body, with those who break the law, with clubs for young people and others, with immigrants—and with all these in their family and social relationships.

Over the past few years opportunities for social work training have grown amazingly. Central and local government departments, organisations of social workers, universities, voluntary bodies and charitable trusts have all helped in this development which within five years has about doubled the number of places in training courses for social work.

Growth of this order is not achieved easily or without risks in work in which high standards are essential; the social worker, whose job is to help people in trouble, must be clear headed about what he is doing and skilful in doing it.

The biggest obstacle to the rapid growth of sound training in social work is, by common consent, the shortage of places in which students can learn to consolidate and extend through practice the knowledge and skills they are acquiring in the classroom and through reading.

There is a shortage of suitable agencies in which students can be trained as well as of competent supervisors, who are the field tutors. Even experienced professional social workers can teach effectively only in an agency which has high standards of practice and where it is understood that the learner must have proper facilities and support if he is to grow in competence. Education for a profession presents problems that are common to law, architecture, engineering, medicine and teaching: how to transmute intellectual comprehension into skilful, effective and imaginative practice.

All the national bodies concerned with the training of social workers have been trying to devise ways in which field placements could be multiplied and used to the best advantage. One necessary step was to get a picture of the current position: how many field work placements were being used? Where were they? Which students were sent to them? What opportunities for expansion and what experiments were being tried? Help from the Gulbenkian Foundation enabled the National Institute for Social Work Training to undertake this first attempt in

Britain to study in a comprehensive way the field work of students as seen by the staff of social work training departments, field work agencies and supervisors, and a small group of students. The survey report indicates the likely increases in demand, identifies new ways for extending field training and for ensuring a rational allocation of places. There was, however, no intention of analysing educational method; this was properly seen as a different task.

The National Institute joins the authors in thanking those who provided the information and the views on which the survey is based; the Gulbenkian Foundation for its generous encouragement and support, including a supplementary grant for publication; the Advisory Committee for wise guidance and the Chairman and Medical Officer of the Public Health Committee of the Buckinghamshire County Council for allowing Miss Gloyne to take part in the survey.

It is difficult to convey the debt owed to Miss Clement Brown and Miss Gloyne. Miss Clement Brown was formerly in charge of the Mental Health Course at the London School of Economics and subsequently Director of Child Care Studies in the Children's Department of the Home Office; Miss Gloyne was Senior Social Worker with the Public Health Department of the Buckinghamshire County Council and came with current experience as a supervisor of students from different types of courses. The survey staff were under no illusion about the difficulty—almost the impossibility—of the task, and they took it on knowing that to be useful it must be done speedily. They have laboured to produce an orderly picture out of a chaotic situation; they have provided evidence where there was little; their report makes clearer what the issues are and where promising new developments lie; it is certain to provoke debate and, we hope, will thus contribute towards more efficient deployment of existing resources and the development of new opportunities in field training on which expanding and improved training for social work must depend.

R. HUWS JONES

CONTENTS

TABLES AND MAPS

TABLES

MAPS

1

THE PICTURE PRESENTED

Purpose of the Survey

In professions concerned with human well-being it is widely accepted that those who qualify need practice as well as study to enable them to gain knowledge, refinement of perception and competence. Most plans of training provide for systematic courses of study combined with skilled teaching or at least experienced guidance for the student while he is engaged in practice. Wide variations exist in the degree of importance attached to each aspect of learning, in timing, and in the ways in which responsibility for teaching is shared and related.

There has been little study in this country of these different patterns,[1] though it is often acknowledged that standards of professional practice are of great importance to social progress.

In education for social work such problems have been discussed since training was pioneered at the beginning of the century by those who recognized it as a skilled service. The issue took on a new significance when courses were designed to meet the needs of particular services, such as medical and psychiatric social work, probation and child care. It was recognized that learning and teaching pursued in hospitals, probation departments or child guidance clinics could be as potent for the eventual wisdom of students as the exercise of thought in tutorials, lectures and libraries. At this stage there came about much more exchange between the staff engaged in both these aspects of learning. A further direction was taken when, partly as the outcome of this exchange, there was more recognition of common knowledge and principles underlying the practice of all social workers.

This Survey was planned for the following main reasons:

1. Recognition that social services called for more qualified social workers.

---

[1] See however, for useful comparisons: Marie Jahoda, *The Education of Technologists; an exploratory case study at Brunel College* Tavistock Publications, 1963.

2. Shortage of suitable field training impeding the setting up of new courses.

3. In courses already established, competition and frustration experienced in making satisfactory arrangements for the practical work and training of an increasing number of students.

Recent developments in training

The past twenty years has seen a series of separate Departmental inquiries into one social service after another. Each report has shewn the need for a substantial increase in the number of social workers competent to give personal service in organizations with widening responsibilities and more exacting standards. Training councils, educational bodies, professional organizations and social work agencies have been making efforts in the face of serious difficulties to provide more and better vocational education.

Two developments mark important stages. The Carnegie Younghusband surveys of the employment and training of social workers[1] led to a demonstration of common principles in all social work, and resulted in the launching of a number of university courses in 'applied social studies', catering for students entering a variety of services.

Secondly, in the *Report of the Working Party on Social Workers in the Local Authority Health and Welfare Services*[2] it was recognized that the universities could not provide a sufficient number of qualified social workers. New courses were set up in educational establishments hitherto unfamiliar with this type of training. The pressure to supply more qualified staff for certain other services, such as child care and probation was at the same time leading to the extension of courses designed particularly to meet these needs. These courses were varied in pattern in the hope of attracting more recruits and of making better use of resources for field work. The issues of quantity and quality, expansion and excellence were encountered at all the cross-roads of social workers, their educators and their employers.

During each of these periods of expansion the hard thinking that had to be done in the shaping of new types of training led in itself to more appraisal of aims and standards.

This particularly affected the staff of social services responsible for

---

[1] Eileen L. Younghusband, *Report on the Employment and Training of Social Workers,* 1947. *Social Work in Britain. A Supplementary Report on the Employment and Training of Social Workers,* 1951. Carnegie United Kingdom Trust, Dunfermline, Fife.
[2] Ministry of Health, *Report of the Working Party on Social Workers in Local Authority Health and Welfare Services.* H.M.S.O., 1959.

the practical work of students. The agencies in which this experience is planned and supervised have thus been exposed simultaneously to many new influences and pressures. At a time when they are faced by acute shortage of staff they have been urged to take more students; to give them a better standard of training; to spend much time deliberating about the aims and methods of new courses; to increase the number of special appointments of student supervisors, and to continue to welcome and to interest students at the beginning of their careers.

It is with the training responsibilities of the staff of social agencies that this study is mainly concerned. It is commonly accepted that satisfactory future developments depend upon the expansion of good opportunities for field work. To bring students to a higher level of wisdom and competence in social services faced with wider responsibilities and already having difficulty in meeting the needs of their clients is indeed a daunting prospect. It was difficult without more comprehensive facts to see how to break away from this enclosing circle of cause and effect.

It would be possible to quote figures from a variety of reports of the extent of the demand for more qualified social workers. We do not propose to do so. This is not only to avoid Parkinson jibes. Such estimates vary and are quickly dated. It can safely be assumed that in the coming decade, if allowances are made for planned increase in establishment, loss of staff and leave of absence for training for those now employed without qualification, there will be need for at least twice the number of trained staff at present employed in casework services alone. Some have placed the figure very much higher. A recent estimate, based upon predictions for a variety of services, was a three-fold increase.[1] Proposals for improving the extent and quality of field work and for easing the burden of those who are responsible for it, can at best achieve only a gradual advance towards this goal. This Survey was undertaken in the hope that this advance might be more purposive and consistent.

Definitions and boundaries

The first question is how to define 'field work'. This is far from simple. The courses for which practical experience is required are not by any means all designed for or undertaken by students who intend to become social workers. Recent studies have shown that there is an increasing tendency for students who graduate in social studies to go

---

[1] Eileen Younghusband, D.B.E., *Social Work Training and Staffing Implications of Community Care*, Social Work, Vol. 22, Nos 2 and 3, April and July 1965, 22–28.

into other types of employment.[1] For such students field work may be arranged in order to enliven their thinking or to help them and their tutors to make up their minds whether social work is their 'line'.

The term 'field work' may be stretched to describe both experience of this kind and also advanced training in the use of knowledge and the refinement of skill.

It would have been simpler and in some ways more satisfactory to concentrate entirely upon the practical training of students who enter a course leading to a recognized qualification for *social work* and to exclude experience in the field arranged for students taking degrees, diplomas or certificates in *social studies*. It was evident however, that such a focus would narrow the scene in two important ways. The staff of social agencies are in fact concerned with students from all types of courses and their responsibilities and difficulties cannot be separated. In many of the services the time and ability of a limited number of staff is divided between students who need highly skilled professional education and those who are only beginning to be aware of how other people live. It was important to find out whether this variety of aims and methods was compatible and achieving satisfactory results. There seemed a possibility either that those who needed specialized teaching were not able to get it because of the claims of other students; or that students of the initial degree and diploma courses might benefit from a wider range of experience if better conditions for their field work could be planned. It was known that interesting experiments were taking place, and it seemed worth while from the point of view of courses, social agencies and students to see whether these might usefully be extended. In addition, from the point of view of individual students proceeding from initial to applied courses, the sequence as well as the nature and quality of experience was of obvious importance.

For all these reasons it was decided to define field work for purposes of the Survey in the following way:

> *Any kind of practical experience in a social organization or agency if this experience has been deliberately arranged for the education of students who are undertaking courses partly or wholly designed for those who intend to become social workers.*

It was necessary to set certain other boundaries to the inquiry and this was done in two ways.

It was decided not to include certain types of kindred training

[1] Barbara N. Rodgers, *The Careers of Social Studies Students*. Occasional Papers on Social Administration, No. 11. The Codicote Press, 1964, p. 19. *University Social Studies Departments Take Stock*, Case Conference, Vol. II, No. 6, November 1964.

different enough to give rise to other kinds of problems. This was held to apply to courses for youth leaders and youth employment officers; for residential work; for personnel officers, or primarily for administrators.

There was a further limitation of an important kind which we were soon compelled to accept. It became apparent that the problem of providing satisfactory field training rested at present mainly with casework services. However important other aspects of social work might be it seemed sensible to start where the recognized need was greatest, and where in fact most of the students were found. The Survey led naturally to the consideration of whether the training in casework agencies was based upon a broad enough study of social need, and whether in professional training as it had been developed in this country, there was too much concentration on personal services and too little upon policy and practice in the development of social resources in the community, or in group work. Already professional courses are being planned along these lines, and it will be seen that recent trends in the field work of students shows some recognition of their importance. In the time at our disposal it was not however possible to do justice to these developments, and we did not include in our detailed inquiries the field work organized, for example, by settlements or community centres or undertaken with groups, in residential establishments or elsewhere. The important and much wider subject of the purpose and scope of university departments of social science and studies and the designation of their students has already received consideration in the valuable studies of Barbara Rodgers and Kathleen Jones.[1][2] It was represented to us by the head of one such department that the university should, for social services, be producing people with a 'questing attitude' and 'attacking minds', alive to many different approaches to social problems. He deplored the fact that students could not at present even *see* skilled practice in fields such as work with groups or in community development. It is to be hoped that further studies along these lines will be encouraged by the questions that emerge from this look at one aspect of social work and the problems of professional education that it presents.

The special programmes of field work arranged in courses particularly designed for overseas students were, reluctantly, not included.

[1] Barbara N. Rodgers, *The Careers of Social Studies Students*. Occasional Papers on Social Administration, No. 11. The Codicote Press, 1964.
[2] Kathleen Jones, *The Teaching of Social Studies in British Universities*. Occasional Papers on Social Administration, No. 12. The Codicote Press, 1964.

Distinction between basic and professional courses

It was necessary to make a broad distinction between two different kinds of courses, and in doing so we followed the terminology of the Joint University Council for Social and Public Administration.[1] The staff concerned with courses leading to a degree, a non-graduate certificate or a graduate diploma in social studies, insist that the word 'training' should not apply to these courses from the point of view of qualifying for social work. Universities offering qualifying courses in this sense have made the difference clear in their title 'Applied Social Studies', or, if the course has a particular focus, by using the name of the service, such as 'Child Care' or 'Medical Social Work'. For the purpose of this inquiry, it was decided to use the word 'basic' for all courses for prospective social workers which did not lead to a qualification recognized for employment by professional organizations and bodies responsible for training, and the word 'professional' for those which were so recognized.

This distinction meant that comprehensive courses of training such as those leading to the Certificate in Social Work which students might enter without having taken any 'basic' course were all grouped as 'professional', though their initial field work might on occasion be akin to that arranged for students of basic courses. To some extent this was arbitrary in terms of practical training. There seemed, however, enough in common between the courses qualifying for employment to justify this broad distinction.

An apology should be made for the use of the word 'professional' partly as a matter of convenience. Pressed into many denotations the currency of this important word is in danger of losing its value. In this context however there is some defence for its use. Much thought is being given to what is implied for social work in the more considered definition of a profession: the sharing of cumulative knowledge and skill between generations and contemporaries, and the standards of personal and social integrity involved. Convergence of interests in organizations of social workers hitherto concerned with particular services and the trend towards 'generic' courses is evidence of growing recognition of common knowledge and principles. This fact is of obvious importance in the future of field work.

Employment following basic courses

The picture is complicated by the fact that although those responsible

---

[1] Joint University Council for Social and Public Administration. *Education for Social Work in the Universities*, J.U.C., 218, Sussex Gardens, London W.2.

for basic courses make it clear that they only *prepare* for professional education and do not provide it, this is by no means always recognized by subsequent employers or by students themselves. In the sellers' market even those with only preliminary courses behind them are at a premium. Barbara Rodgers in the already quoted study[1] shows that while rather more than half the university students undertaking social study courses eventually proceed to professional training, only about a third do so without an interval during which they may or may not be employed as social workers. Academic staff responsible for basic courses sometimes find themselves bound to recognize this in arranging the field work for their students, and it has added to the confusion of some of the social agencies about the kind of practical experience and training which should be given. They may be faced with the fact that some of these students have already been appointed to a responsible post at the time they undertake practical work. This situation is pertinent to the Survey.

Theory and practice

It is commonly accepted that professional competence involves the integration of knowledge with personal skill. It may be asked therefore whether it is profitable to separate the consideration of what and how students are expected to gain in the field, from their learning in the class room and the library. It may well be shown that this is indeed an artificial separation, and if so perhaps one of the most important purposes of the Survey will be achieved. Although the lecture, seminar or tutorial may be regarded as primarily an intellectual approach to discovery and logical discipline, even so-called academic learning must be based to some extent on the living experience of the student and this influences his freedom to entertain new knowledge and ideas. Similarly, the social work supervisor choosing and discussing certain kinds of experience must be concerned with the student's knowledge and capacity for clear conceptual thought as well as with his responses to people and his practical capabilities. The usual words 'theory' and 'practice' suggest an unreal distinction in the process of learning, as though something were picked up in one place and put down in another. The important difference lies between a live situation in which the student is in action and one in which his pursuit of knowledge and experiments in ideas are for the time being protected from immediate demands and consequences. It is trite to say that concepts and principles emerge from experience as well as from study. Sometimes, however,

[1] See p. 14, footnote.

it seems that the need for intelligent thought in the practice of social work is curiously under-rated. A report by a university teacher on a graduate contemplating professional training for social work ran 'Although her heart is in social work she has none the less shown some ability in abstract ideas'.

In the planning of training there are always problems in helping students to relate these two approaches to learning. In the nature of things they are as a rule physically, if not psychologically, separated. Some maintain that unity can only be preserved if the same teacher is concerned with both, and in social work this has often been contrived by appointments shared between agency and college, or by university staff taking responsibility for teaching in the field. In the training of teachers the staff of training colleges normally take considerable responsibility for supervising the class-room teaching of students in schools, though there is indication that more reliance is likely to be placed upon practising teachers.[1] In the medical profession the clinical teaching of students is in the hands of gifted practitioners. There are different views of great interest about the best ways of combining the advantages on the one hand of close identification with the situation in which the profession is practised and on the other, the integration of verbal and practical learning. One question that arises, for example, is whether a different kind of educational skill is involved in teaching based upon 'live' experience.

Variety in practice and in opinion is illustrated in the training of social workers at the present time. In professional courses there is increasing tendency for field work to be carried on concurrently with study and in near-by agencies. This is partly because of the belief that in this way students themselves hold the two in more effective relation, and partly because it is thought that better educational methods will follow from close partnership of the staff. On the other hand a large number of students undertake full-time periods of field work, sometimes at a distance from their courses. This plan also has its adherents on the grounds of better concentration on each kind of learning and more identification with the service. It would be of great interest to study the outcome of these different methods in terms of the achievements of students, but this is outside the scope of this Survey. The views of the staff and the practical effects of these different patterns are however explored since they are central to the development of training in the future.

[1] Ministry of Education, *Half Our Future: A report of the Central Advisory Council for Education* (England). H.M.S.O. 1963. Chapter 12.

Groups of students in field work

A student undertaking field work in a social agency may be placed singly or may find himself with a number of others from different courses according to the nature and scale of the service. If he is with others there are varieties of plans, from individual supervision to a special programme of teaching for a group, often called a 'student unit', in charge of a member of staff appointed for this purpose. Groups of this kind are being extended and are of particular interest both from the educational standpoint and also because they are one means of increasing the opportunities for practical training.

Enough has been said to show that the selection of field work for special study does not imply that in terms of education it is separable from other aspects of learning. The Survey, for good reasons, has not been concerned with the content of study courses or the manner of their teaching, but it has naturally been of interest to discover whether there is reciprocity between the staff responsible for students in the field and those by whom they are taught in colleges, and whether students themselves think there is useful relationship between their experiences in study and in practice.

The changing scene

Even in the twelve months during which facts and opinions were assembled, we sometimes felt like the old advertisement of the disappearing car 'That's Shell . . . that *was*!' Each year training councils and educational bodies were considering different patterns of training. New courses were starting, sometimes in colleges unfamiliar with this type of training. The social agencies in surrounding areas were being explored and cultivated with a view to field work. Fresh devices were being contrived for attracting older students, for training the employed but unqualified, and for providing in-service programmes of study. Moreover, apart from these developments there is almost no pause in the succession of students. This continues like a constantly revolving turnstile. Applications for the following year must be considered while present students are being introduced; new students may arrive while reports on their predecessors are still in the pipe-line. In the nature of things, it is difficult to find any interval when experiences may be carefully weighed and policy determined. The impetus of change is both an added reason and an almost insuperable difficulty for a survey of this kind. Facts were necessarily out-of-date almost before they could be committed to paper.

Nevertheless, 'stills' from strips of film are sometimes a good example of their quality. Changes often reflect the permanence of problems and principles. A study of the recent past may throw some light on the shape of things to come, if only by raising provocative questions.

A true measure of the quality of training depends upon how well human needs are met by the social services designed to provide them. In this study it was only possible to get a picture of the aims and methods of training within the services as they are at present. Furthermore the Survey was not intended as a study of the outcome of different methods of training. All that has been attempted is to report the facts of an extensive programme, the views on certain main issues of those who are taking part in it, the compatability of various aims and methods, and to record experiments which may have useful bearing upon developments in the future.

Methods of the Survey

Readers who prefer first to have a complete description of the methods used rather than the brief account which follows should now turn to the Appendix (p. 135).

The Survey was based upon facts assembled about field work undertaken during the twelve months from 1 October 1962 to 30 September 1963.

There were four main sources of information: the academic staff in charge of courses in which any practical work was included; the social workers in agencies where students were received for field work during this period (now called 'the Survey year'); professional organizations of social workers, and a small group of students.

Correspondence inquiries were sent to all the staff in charge of courses in the United Kingdom and Eire. The first called for the main facts about field work in the Survey year; the second for opinions about some of the chief issues which came to light in interviews.

In two areas interviews were held with the staff in charge of local courses and of all the agencies in which students had been received. In a third area, chosen because comparatively few students were sent there, discussions were held with the staff of a number of organizations possibly suitable for the training of students, in addition to those in which students had been received. Interviews were also held with the staff of courses and certain agencies providing for a large number of students, and a special study was made of 'student units'. The views of the staff of agencies receiving students in some primarily rural areas at a distance from courses were invited by correspondence.

Professional associations of social workers and organizations of

senior officers of certain services were invited to comment upon some
of the main issues emerging from these inquiries. An organization of
present students assembled the views of members.

The findings of a similar Survey in Scotland, carried out by the
Scottish Home and Health Department after consultation, is combined
with other evidence in the report which follows.

SEQUENCE OF CHAPTERS

In the next chapter all sources of evidence are used in describing the
characteristic aims and methods of field work for students in basic and
professional courses.

Chapters 3 and 4 are concerned first with the ways in which decisions
are reached by the staff of courses and of agencies in the choice of field
work, and then with the nature of their partnership.

In Chapter 5 attention is given to the teaching arrangements made
in certain agencies for groups of students, referred to as 'student units'.

Chapter 6 deals with methods by which field work is being or might
be expanded.

The concluding Chapter 7 contains interpretations of all the findings
and suggestions for future developments, summarized in the final
pages.

2

AIMS AND METHODS IN FIELD WORK

IF educational practice is essential for becoming a competent social worker, aims and methods must be the joint concern of those who arrange field work for their students and those by whom it is supervised. In this chapter the main purposes expressed or implied on both sides and the methods most commonly used will be described. The choice of particular kinds of field work and the nature of the partnership between academic and social work staff will then be discussed in the light of what they hope will be achieved.

A distinction has already been made between the use of the terms 'basic' and 'professional' courses. The classified list (Table IA and IB pp. 42 and 43) provides further definition. There is another important difference between the professional courses which include field work. Some offer a complete sequence of study and practice without requiring the student first to have taken a basic course; others involve for students two separate programmes often in different colleges, the first basic, the second applied, or professional. The picture is further complicated in two ways: first by the fact that not all students undertaking basic courses intend to become social workers, and second, because those who enter the social services may be employed without taking professional training. All these facts affect aims and methods of field work.

Aims were discussed with the academic and social work staff, and their views were also invited in writing. It must be recognized that in training, as in many other pursuits, aims are often implicit and identified only as methods are analysed. Ideas were sometimes given off the cuff in interviews; others were the result of careful deliberation, sometimes expressed in published or written statements apart from the inquiries of the survey.

There was striking contrast between the clearness of purpose and mutual understanding of social workers and academic staff in the basic and professional courses. Even when differences between the needs of the students were recognized by field work staff, the nature of these differences and the way in which they should determine the experiences and supervision of students in the field was often far from clear. This was partly because communication between the academic staff and the agencies in the basic courses were tenuous and often haphazard, as later chapters will show. In contrast a great deal of face to face discussion about the educational experience of students took place between the staff in most of the professional courses. When students from both types of courses were received in one agency there was apt to be confusion of aims and methods.

This confusion was found in many of the casework agencies, where the large majority of students from both types of course were placed in the Survey year. In other settings, such as Settlements, to which a number of students go from basic courses, and which unfortunately were not included in the Survey, there might have been a clearer picture of the aims and methods of training for students at this stage.

However, apart from residential work, by far the largest proportion of all student placements of at least four weeks, whether from basic or from professional courses were in the casework services, and these mainly concentrated in certain public and voluntary agencies. (See Tables IIA and IIB, pp. 44 and 45). Within the public services (Table IIA p. 44) over three-quarters of all the student placements are either in children's departments, medical social work or probation. If mental health services are added this accounts for over 95 per cent. In the first three there is a close similarity between the proportions in each service of all the basic course students and all the professional students. There is a difference in the extent to which voluntary agencies are used for students from the two types of course; 87 per cent of the total number of placements of students from professional courses are in publicly supported services compared with 59 per cent of students from basic courses; but in the voluntary agencies too, far the largest proportion of both groups are placed in those providing family casework (Table IIB, p. 45). Looking only at the total number of students from basic courses, 71 per cent of placements of any kind, apart from those in residential work, were in casework services:

It seems therefore justifiable to pay special attention to what happens to both groups of students in this setting, and to ask what it is hoped they will achieve, and by what means.

PART I

BASIC COURSES

Length of field work

The total amount of time given to field work by students in all kinds of basic courses throughout the period of their study varied between six and twenty-six weeks. The widest variation was in degree courses. In some of these field work is only arranged after graduation 'if required'. In others the number of weeks is widely scattered between the two extremes quoted above. This disparity in itself implies widely differing views about its function.

There seems more unanimity in the post-graduate one year courses, in which the large majority of students undertake between twelve and sixteen weeks of field work. In the two-year non-graduate courses the usual total length of time in the field is between fourteen and twenty weeks.[1] Almost all the students undertake field work in block periods of varied length during the vacations.

Students from basic courses commonly spend eight weeks in any one casework agency. By the time they have this experience most of them will have seen something at first hand of social conditions and activities in Settlements or industry, youth clubs or local authority departments. Many of them now spend some weeks in residence, the majority with children. (See Table III, p. 105.)

Aims of field work

Much discussion in the Joint University Council for Social and Public Administration and elsewhere has centred round the aims of field work for students in social study courses. Many diverse requests are received by the agencies, but there seems seldom to have been any attempt on the part of field workers and academic staff to think out together what learning is likely to result from particular kinds of experience.

The London Family Welfare Association, training a large number of students from various courses, listed twenty-seven different ideas in the communications they received about individual students, of which the following are illustrations.[2]

---

[1] Kathleen Jones, *A Review of University Social Studies Departments.* University of Manchester, 1963. Appendix IA. pp. 14–16.

[2] Reproduced by kind permission of the Family Welfare Association, Denison House, Vauxhall Bridge Road, S.W.1.

A final linking up of theory and practice and clarification of problems facing families and the services for helping them. If a student is helped to see what casework methods are, she will I think develop an ability to use this method of helping fruitfully.

This student needs an all-round experience of general family case-work agency work. She also needs to begin to interview and visit on her own and should be able to do this by now. She is not yet at the stage when she could undertake intensive work with a few families and should therefore be placed where she could get a wide variety and where her main work will be offering services rather than skilled help with personal problems.

An introduction to casework, an opportunity to accept responsibility for helping people in social need, contact with a fairly wide range of families and services, an opportunity to note the differences in approach between the nurse and the social worker, an opportunity to learn something of the casework skills as a background to a more professional training, an opportunity to study the factors other than psychological which contribute towards social breakdown, a contact with a fairly wide range of cases, an opportunity to see how different social services co-operate together.

Such diverse and comprehensive aims, even if their fulfilment were practicable, seem to call for intimate knowledge by tutors as well as supervisors of the kinds of experience that could'be offered and their likely outcome.

In the aims expressed by the academic staff during the Survey there were four main constellations of ideas about what they hoped would be provided in field work:

(a) A means whereby students can test their liking for the work and the staff can judge their capacities.

(b) Providing illustration or illumination of what is being learned in other ways.

(c) Administrative aspects: gaining knowledge of the purposes and organization of social services.

(d) Personal experience with individuals and families in need and ways of helping them.

A test of suitability for social work

(a) The first of these aims held good particularly for degree students who might or might not be entering social work and were therefore using this experience partly as a sample of a career. For those who had passed this stage it was the other three purposes to which reference was most commonly made. At the receiving end, this wide diversity of aims even if they were understood, was bewildering. The same agency may be asked to carry out plans for students who are not yet sure what they want to learn and for those who expect, and are indeed sometimes expected to 'do' casework.

Providing illustrations

(b) Academic staff regarded practised observation and pertinent illustrations of their studies as one of the most important purposes of learning in the field at this stage. Reference was made to two purposes of observation, one focused on the way in which experienced social workers helped people in need and the other on the organization of agencies designed for this and for kindred services. This kind of purpose was described by a tutor responsible for post-graduate students:

> Classroom teaching on social administration too easily suggests that Acts of Parliament create changes and it is only by field experience that the student learns that change is a continuing process in which Acts are merely milestones.

Another description of this kind came from a university where only a small proportion of degree students were preparing for social work:

> Field work is primarily undertaken for the research project which is a requirement of the course. . . . Topics covered by field work are not limited to social work agencies and in fact a comparatively small proportion of students chose this type of subject. Frequently it is chosen by those intending to make social work their career and here observation of the social services has an additional purpose as field work.

The following comment was made by a university teacher in response to an invitation to give her views on a number of aims commonly expressed in the Survey interviews. Referring to the aim *practical illustrations of what is taught and discussed in lectures and classes*, she wrote:

> This is of special importance if you mean using field work experience for social study as a scientist uses laboratory work in systematic study, but it seems to me that this would mean more time and

more organization than is given to this side of the work at present and that we have got no distance at all towards achieving this aim.

The difficulty has been expressed by some university teachers in an unpublished document:[1]

> Practice can illuminate theory and theory practice, provided that practice is an integral part of the course respected by all who teach it. The challenge for practical work in Departments of Social Study is to organize it better and prepare for it and follow it up more carefully.

Mere unsystematized looking may, it is suggested, leave the student 'bored, frustrated and rebellious'.

Professor Donnison has written:[2]

> If students are helped to identify problems for special study, if they read about them and are able—whether through practical work or formal research—to examine these problems under appropriate supervision, and if they have to report their finding at some length in a form that can be academically assessed, then the field studies required of students of social administration can make a real contribution to university education. They are a reminder to teachers and students alike that social scientists are concerned with the real world.

Contact with social workers who enjoy what they are doing and who think it worth while is in itself valued by tutors when they consider its first impact upon students; this generating of interest and enthusiasm was thought by one tutor to be the most important value of early experience. For students who have gone further and who are spending important years in systematic study 'illumination' must surely involve more than this. Yet evidence in the agencies showed that although supervisors were often aware that experience should illustrate theory, they seldom knew enough of the student's academic work to understand *what* should be illustrated. 'Observation' was an accepted purpose; this seemed in casework agencies to consist of a rather general introduction to the neighbourhood; of watching the cross-roads in the office, being present at staff interviews, and attending certain meetings. The academic staff assumed responsibility for helping students to find 'illustrations' and for discussing, after their experience, its possible

---

[1] From the introduction to a Field Work Manual in preparation by the Field Work Sub-Committee of the Social Administration Committee of the Joint University Council for Social and Public Administration, 1964.

[2] D. V. Donnison, *The Teaching of Social Administration*, The British Journal of Sociology, Vol. XII, No. 3, 1961, p.203.

relation to their studies. From the point of view of the staff of the agency, this is essentially a 'one way' relationship, as we shall see in later chapters. There seemed a large element of chance in what was hoped for these students and what was likely to happen.

Knowledge of the administration of social services

(c) To study the administration of a service is sometimes part of a field work project set by the university, and may be carried out in local government departments as well as in casework agencies. One example given by a university teacher of this kind of 'administrative case-study' was to help the student to learn 'the process of decision taking'. Barbara Butler described one of her aims for post-graduate students to learn 'the immediate functions of the agency, and the way in which it fits or avoids fitting in with other agencies'. She adds that it is also important for them to understand the 'administrative pattern' and efficient office practice.[1] This aim seemed generally to be accepted by those in the field. The Scottish survey stated that supervisors felt their first responsibility to basic course students was 'to show a social agency in action and to indicate something of its relationship with other agencies and the kinds of problems which come its way'.

Much trouble is taken in the agencies to introduce students to a variety of committees and conferences showing the process of administration. This experience might raise useful questions about such problems as 'the process of decision taking' if skilled educational guidance were given. There were instances of good preparation of students for attendance at meetings, by description of the functions of members and explanation of items on the agenda.

Experience of serving individuals in need

(d) Almost all the academic staff look to field work to help students to learn about people and the way they live. One expressed it 'To discover what is normal to daily living beyond the range of one's own upbringing'. By some this is seen as going considerably further than mere 'knowing'. Widening their experience of individuals and families with unfamiliar attitudes and traditions is seen as an important means of beginning to gain insight, an exercise in what might be called 'hearing their own accents'. This experience may contribute towards 'maturity' so often said to be the aim for students, but seldom defined. It was this point of view which was urged in support of taking them out

[1] Barbara Butler, *The Two Months' Placement for Social Studies Students*, Case Conference, Vol. 8, No. 2, June 1961, pp. 35–38.

of the local climate of their own upbringing or education. Others saw particular value in students assuming an unfamiliar role outside the framework of social services, such as employment in a factory, hospital ward or cafe; this is often recommended before students enter college. Direct experience with their neighbours in Settlements and community centres was seen in part as adding to knowledge about and tolerance of variety in people and circumstances.

In casework agencies academic staff hoped that students would begin to understand the kind of problems brought to social workers and that they would be given a measure of responsibility for offering help of a practical kind. Here there were confusions and misunderstandings about reasonable aims for beginners. It was the view of some of the university staff that young or inexperienced students were sometimes taken out of their depth by social workers who expected them to benefit from the same methods that they used with students at the professional stage. Others lamented the fact that students were not given enough to do. The first of these risks was expressed some years ago by Katharine Lloyd:

> Often in the past there has been an attempt to 'water down' professional knowledge and administer it in small doses. There is some danger that this may in a sense immunise the student against real professional learning.[1]

This risk seems still to be felt. Some academic staff emphasized the view that it was important at an early stage not to interfere with the student's spontaneity, compassion and common sense, whereas supervisors thought that from the outset students should by means of discussion, begin to gain insight into the ways in which their own needs and prejudices might impinge upon their ability to meet those of other people. One university teacher with long experience of the supervision of students, deplored too much discussion of their personal attitudes at this stage and said that they should not be discouraged from 'identifying' with people in trouble; she hoped that when they first went to casework agencies they would find that they liked and were interested in people and that above all they would learn to respect them. Summarizing the views of supervisors of students from these courses in Scotland is the comment 'students were not expected to have much insight, but to be beginning to think imaginatively about people'.

Individual differences between students are obviously of great

[1] A. K. Lloyd, *Field Work as part of Undergraduate Preparation for Professional Education*, The Social Service Review, Chicago, Vol. XXX, No. 1, March 1956.

importance in this controversy. Certain fundamental principles of adult education are also involved. What is likely to prove a fruitful sequence of learning in the experience of human relationships? Does discussion of subjective attitudes detract from, or rightly handled, add to interest in and feeling for individuals? These questions in relation to students in basic courses seem to be the subject of argument rather than joint study and consultation.

Methods used in the agencies

The methods used with students in the field showed very varied interpretations of aims. Supervisors often said that they were planning their work with little awareness of what the students were learning in other ways. These difficulties seldom affected the welcome they were given, of which there was evidence in personal introduction to individual members of the staff. The majority of students felt that the staff were glad to have them, as indeed they generally were.

The reading of case records is a common method of introducing students to the service. From the comments of students this has diminishing returns, and is possibly over-used because of the difficulty for busy staff of devising a balanced programme. Some supervisors recognized the limited value of this method; one expressed the view that such reading could only be of much benefit to experienced social workers. The danger, without focus and activity, of becoming 'bored, frustrated and rebellious' was vividly illustrated by some of the students:

> I needed a chance to prove I could meet and talk to clients—to give me self-confidence. The officer realized this and did the best she could in what she considered to be too short a period for cases of my own. Too much time spent idling in the general office reading case notes of people I hadn't met.
> (Aged 22. Certificate in Social Study, First year. 4 weeks period.)

> Was not allowed to come in contact with clients or attend interviews, and had to spend a large amount of time alone with just books.
> (Aged 21, Certificate in Social Study, First year.)

> I was bored most of the time. One reaches saturation point quickly (at least at this level) and one can only pine to do something oneself.
> (Aged 27. Basic course, Second year. 8 weeks period.)

A more lively way of learning, but with its own complications, is listening to interviews. This bears some resemblance to the training of medical students and is one way of reconciling responsibility for client and student if it is supported by skilled teaching. Reference was often made to golden opportunities to discuss shared interviews in car journeys. One supervisor said that he encouraged students to criticize his records, and used these journeys to discuss with the student how to record the interview.

It was generally recognized both that it was of value for students to take some independent responsibility and also that they should have the satisfaction of doing something useful which was not likely to lead to personal complications. Here there were problems, partly because of unpredictable events, and partly because of differences of view. In a number of agencies however ingenuity is used in devising 'safe' and useful services for inexperienced students, such as escorting children or visiting well established foster homes. Some students are sometimes well aware of the difficulty of the staff in judging what they are able to undertake—for example:

> I was given to understand that my placements were to be pre-liminary case work, but I felt the work to be more advanced than this, and had it not been for very helpful supervision I should have been overwhelmed.
> (Aged 38. Certificate in Social Study, Second year.)

Judgement of the stage reached by individuals is not easy even with much knowledge about their experience and capabilities: those who supervise students from basic courses often do not have this knowledge. On the other hand the experienced caseworker must in the nature of things be the person to assess the difficulties with which a student is or may be faced. More often than not academic staff have not recently had experience of this kind in the field, and it may be difficult for them to judge its impact on the student and the best use of educational opportunities. Reflections about this difficulty are made in some of the comments of the professional associations later in this chapter. Misunderstandings can be spread by students who are too easily thrown by their experiences, or quickly excited by new discoveries, and who may dramatize their impressions as they pass from agency to college. This calls for the closest mutual understanding on the part of supervisors and tutors which, in basic courses, is rarely established.

Case records

The importance of learning to write useful records is recognized on both sides, but there is great variety in the way these records are used for educational purposes. Some students, even at this early stage in their field work are expected to make long reports of interviews so that they can be used for discussion with their supervisors; others did not appear even to consult regularly with the staff about the content and arrangement of the reports that went into the files.

Supervision

The evidence of present students illustrated different practices in discussion of their work. In the replies of 99 students in basic courses about half said that they had regular weekly or more frequent discussions, somewhat over a quarter talks when there was time and occasion. About one in every five commented that they had very little supervision indeed. The following illustrations show very different experiences. One student expressed great appreciation of the qualities of her supervisor, but said she was too busy for discussion, and wrote:

> Time is precious and one was inclined to be left sitting in empty offices reading old copies of The *Almoner* or books on almoning, psychology, etc.
>
> (Aged 21. Non-graduate two year course; 1st year.)

Others said:

> We discussed social work and its very varied aspects and difficulties just about all the time we were not actually interviewing or on visits. I learned a great deal from my supervisor, but what I learned was not 'casework' it was more the inadequacy of casework and general principles of social work.
>
> (Age 23. Non-graduate two year course; 2nd year.)

> One period of discussion with the senior officer after six weeks and another at the end. General and complete lack of supervision. Was left for many hours on my own with nothing to do.
>
> (Aged 22. Degree course; 3rd year.)

Reports on students

Reports on the field work of students, for which outlines are often sent to the agencies, are generally expected by tutors. These reports may be one of the most important means of communication between the staff of agencies and courses, and as such will be further considered in Chapter 3. They may also be a method of education if they are used for discussion of their progress with students. Some tutors ask that this should be done. There seems however to be great variety of practice. In the answers given by present students in 100 placements to a question about the discussion of their reports, half had not discussed them with their supervisors, and in a third of the placements it was said that there had been no discussion with supervisor or tutor. Failure to discuss reports with students in the agency may again show uncertainty about aims and achievements. One student wrote, perhaps reflecting staff uncertainty as well as her own:

> I should very much like to have had a final session with my supervisor to discuss what I had learned and whether I had made any progress during this period. It is very difficult to assess one's own progress, especially when one is not sure in which direction one is supposed to be progressing.

Basic Courses: Summary and Implications

Very considerable use is made of casework agencies for students from basic courses, and there is much good will in receiving them. Lack of clearness of purpose for students from different types of course leads to empirical methods in their practical experience which is seldom closely related to the other aspects of the students' learning. Methods of teaching casework suitable for professional students are sometimes employed for those regarded by academic staff as unprepared for this experience; other educational needs are often not well met because of lack of understanding between academic and field work staff, and of staff time.

There is evidence of concern about these problems on the part of some academic staff; statements about general and specific purposes are being drafted. Other types of field work related more closely to studies might provide for some students better alternatives to casework. Field workers and academic staff need to consider together aims, opportunities and methods.

PART II

PROFESSIONAL COURSES

The relation between the staff of agencies and of most of the professional courses presents a very different picture. The contrast is more striking, since these students were also coming from a wide variety of courses, some generic and some catering for particular services; some offering comprehensive and others only 'applied' training following

C

basic courses; some arranging concurrent and some block periods of theory and practice. It will be seen later that there were marked differences in the closeness of the partnership. Nevertheless, the central concern of the staff of professional courses stands out as much more clear and consistent. Put in its most simple terms, students are sent to and received by casework agencies to learn how to be of help to people. It is to the supervisors of field work that the academic staff look to develop the student's ability to understand people's difficulties and to become capable of constructive professional service in this sense.

To be able to give this help is seen largely as dependent upon their skill in personal relationships. It is generally accepted that the ability to serve the needs of other people involves insight into the ways in which the social workers' own attitudes affect what is called 'objectivity' or 'disinterestedness', a concept also involved in 'maturity'. To have insight into their own attitudes and to be able to tolerate in other people such attitudes as hostility or dependency is widely seen as essential in the development of professional responsibility. There was little direct reference to the discernment of different kinds of needs and social resources, a concept essential to social diagnosis, probably because this was seen as inherent in satisfactory professional relations. Academic staff and supervisors considered it important that personal service should be seen in relation to the function of the agency and the organization by which it was provided, but their methods implied a less clear grasp of how this balance of aims might be achieved.

Occasionally it seems that more thought is given to the quality of professional relationship than to the ends it serves. Some saw the danger that this might be so, and urged that the purpose of professional training should be seen as 'diagnosis for social *work*' rather than preoccupation with the psychology of the individual. It was our impression that the joint discussions between field workers and academic staff, at first greatly concerned with a changing emphasis in meeting personal needs, were leading to clearer definition and perspective. A significant remark was made by a supervisor that whereas students of basic courses, apparently affected by esoteric ideas about the social worker, sometimes 'wanted to do *deep* casework', those in professional courses had 'got beyond this stage'.

Changing perspective is shown by realization of the importance of group relationships instanced in the growing value placed upon residential work and in other ways. Many questions were also being raised about the best ways of helping students to get a sound grasp of the administration of social services.

Field work and study are generally seen as two ways of approaching coherent learning, though this is much more true when both are undertaken concurrently, as later chapters will show. This presents a contrast to the one way relationship in basic courses, in which field work experience tends to be seen as a means to the educational purposes of the academic staff. In the professional courses it is assumed that the students go to the agency to learn by taking increasing responsibility and that in this they will be supported by their academic study of human development and relationships and the principles of casework, the social services and their sanctions.

Methods are naturally affected by the length and concentration of field work. The proportion of full time, 'block' placements in all professional courses was 56 per cent, and of part-time, carried on concurrently with study 44 per cent. In some courses one period of field work was full time and another concurrent. A few courses in which large numbers of students were trained accounted for most of the block placements. Full time field work was for not less than three months, occasionally for four months and exceptional instances were given of a five month period. Concurrent field work was typically arranged for three days a week (occasionally two), over a period of four to five months, and in the university courses was often completed by some weeks full time.

The large majority of supervisors interviewed who were able to compare the two plans regarded concurrent training as providing more satisfactory methods of learning and teaching. This view was essentially related to the closer partnership with academic staff characteristic of this type of course and considered in Chapter 4. The staff saw advantages in the longer period the students had for developments in casework and in their own opportunities for preparation, but their main argument was the closer relation between practice and theory brought about for them and for the students.

Some of the staff providing courses in which block field work was adopted and some of their supervisors maintained that this plan brought about for the students a closer identification with the service, and that they then learned more effectively. They stressed the importance of students being available for all the vicissitudes of their clients and able to attend Court sessions and other important meetings. In these agencies there tended to be more insistence that the students should become familiar with all the procedures of the service and get a thorough grasp of legal sanctions and their interpretation. This emphasis was affected by the fact that most of the students placed for full time field work were preparing for employment in the agency in which they were being trained. In the Scottish report it was found that rather more than half the supervisors preferred block to concurrent training. It was however stated that the small group of supervisors who were professionally trained and had had considerable experience saw more advantage in concurrent placements 'because of their value for the even progress of theoretical and practical training, side by side, throughout the period of the course'.

Learning about administration

It was often stated that all students should gain knowledge of administrative responsibilities, but there was much less confidence and consistency in the methods by which this should be achieved than there was in the teaching of casework. It was difficult to tell how far in dis-cussion of their cases administrative implications were considered. In small and less complex organizations there was sometimes little reference to this aspect of their work. In certain large agencies there was also found a lack of contact between the supervisors and responsible administrators in interpreting policy and organization. Teaching of this kind was more highly developed in hospitals where student units were established (see Chapter 5). In some local authority services there have been experiments in special programmes for students at head-quarters offices where the policy and organization was described by the head of the department and members of the administrative staff talked about their responsibilities, which were illustrated as the students spent part of the day with them.

There have been other projects in professional courses designed for students to make a special study of the administration of a variety of social agencies. In a course for experienced students leading to the Certificate in Social Work it was found after experiment that it was more productive to set students to work in groups on the study of certain kinds of human need and with the help of visits and reports to describe and compare the organizations designed to meet these needs than it was to spend time in agencies for the study of administration as such.

Learning and teaching casework

Certain methods of teaching casework to students from professional courses are widely adopted. In their initial introductions and in the plans for their full participation the staff supervising their work show willingness from the outset to give them a share of responsibility. The welcome the students received was evident in the comments of staff and students. 'We felt as though the fatted calf had been killed' said one group of their reception.

The main medium for learning and teaching is for a small number of carefully chosen cases to be entrusted to the student after consultation, and for their own account of interviews to form the basis of educational discussion to which regular weekly time is given. There is an interesting contrast here with the methods of supervising the practice of student teachers who are usually seen in action by the staff for discussion of methods.

Students begin to take this responsibility after a relatively short introduction to case records. Much thought is given to the choice of cases in relation to the experience and capabilities of individuals. They are often entrusted with new applications to the agency as well as with clients already familiar to the staff. Methods of interviewing are then central to their learning and are prepared and reviewed in consultation with the supervisor. Very full accounts (known as 'process recording') of what happened between client and student is encouraged by academic staff and used by most supervisors as a basis for these discussions. It is however recognized by tutors as well as supervisors that the educational value of discussing detailed records of the to and fro of an interview depends upon the confidence of the staff and their skill. Students are expected to differentiate between these records used for educational purposes and those which the service requires, for which they are, naturally, also responsible.

Discussion involving personal attitudes of interviewer and client tends by its nature to lead to a relationship with the supervisor of particular importance to the student. Careful thought was being given in some of the joint meetings of field workers and academic staff to the distinction between attitudes of the student which have an inevitable bearing upon professional capabilities and those which are only of personal concern. Some supervisors and students thought that discussion in groups was a useful method of keeping perspective in this personal way of learning. This was one of the arguments in favour of student units.

Most supervisors and professional organizations give support to this 'slow motion' method of learning casework. Some striking educational advances were reported in concurrent courses when discoveries in study and in experience merged and were explored both with tutor and supervisor. There are however some differences of view about the degree of concentration on a few cases, bearing in mind the need to adapt to later pressures of employment. It was generally recognized that the pace should be quickened and the range widened during the final stages of training. Some supervisors were well aware that this balance was needed, but still emphasized the educational value of intensive rather than extensive experience. For example:

> At one time a student could have six or seven cases; twelve cases in a placement where they (the students) have developed quite a way would be enough. 'Slow motion' training may present difficulties on the job, but one should not sacrifice this opportunity of learning because of this. Students could not do intensive work study with the kind of load which is normal in the field.

and again

> They have to be made to stop and think about each case. A good case must be an academic exercise. There is need for these students to take a step at a time, but they get there in the end.

Occasionally we encountered in senior members of the staff some exasperation at the degree of consideration and protection that was given to students:

> Students are given too much attention and are too sheltered from the job; they expect to be V.I.P.s; they should do a job as soon as possible.

Views of professional associations

Evidence on the teaching of casework and its relation to other aspects of social service was given by five professional associations of social workers. Their opinions were invited upon the following statement:

Preparation of students for responsibilities in employment

Some staff regard 'slow motion' casework on very few cases as essential to satisfactory learning during professional training. According to this view well-trained students quickly acquire special knowledge about the agency in which they become employed. Others are troubled if students are not required to gain specific knowledge of certain agencies and to adapt themselves to particular administrative and other pressures during their training.

Reservations made by professional associations to their general approval of this method of teaching were mainly in the difficulty of achieving a balance between casework skill and a sound grasp of the administrative responsibilities of the agency. This provides further confirmation of other evidence, and is illustrated in the following extracts from replies:

> Slow motion and small caseloads are essential to learning during the early part of professional teaching so that firm foundations can be laid. The teaching of facts particular to the agency and the caseworker's place in it can be done in such a way that they are seen as illustrations of general concepts and principles which will apply in other settings. There should be a stepping up of caseloads in the second placement and towards the end the student should be able to take 'unselected' referrals. She should also be able to establish priorities and have some sense of urgency and responsibility in her work. The timing of this may vary greatly from one student to another.
>
> (Institute of Medical Social Workers, Education Committee.)
>
> There seemed to be no reason why students doing 'slow motion' casework (implying casework without pressure, giving time to consider, discuss and record fully) should not, at the same time, acquire knowledge of the agency in which they are training. . . . As casework is a method of help employed by certain agencies in order that they should efficiently carry out their prescribed functions, casework practice has little meaning without due regard for, and an understanding of social policy and administrative procedures of specific agencies. While it was not thought necessary for the student to have a detailed knowledge of the administration of a setting they should learn enough to be able to adapt their work to particular fields.
>
> (Association of Family Case Workers.)
>
> We would stress that students should always be kept aware of a whole case, its legal implications and the statutory or departmental policy authorizing the worker's actions, the administrative procedures involved, as well as the personal needs of the client and the casework aspects to be considered. . . . Examples were cited (i.e. by their members) of beginning workers who had been trained by 'slow motion' casework and thereby had become divorced from social purpose and agency function. It is suggested that students should work very hard on a few cases—not too few. Students need to feel under pressure but the pressure should not be from the number of cases but from the work being done on a few cases.
>
> (Association of Child Care Officers.)

It was clear that all members thought 'slow motion' learning on a few cases was essential to their professional training and that such method of teaching deepened their insight and gave them confidence in their skill. All worked under much greater pressure in their first job, but they thought the experience during training of working in a protected setting with high standards, gave them a standard to aim at in their work, and enabled them to adapt to the demands of the job.

(Association of Psychiatric Social Workers.)

In general newly qualified workers returning to departments have been satisfied that casework training on a very few cases has prepared them for subsequent employment. When they take up employment, professional supervision (in the sense of an experienced and qualified officer whom they can consult) would be of general advantage.

(County Welfare Officers Society.)

The value of continued supervision in the first year of employment was also stressed by the National Association of Probation Officers.

Two Associations of senior officers—the Association of Directors of Welfare Services and the Association of Children's Officers also endorsed the view that 'slow motion' casework was essential to learning, and, in agreement with many of the comments, that towards the end of the course they should begin to experience the pressing claims of casework and administration involved in employment.

Reports on students

This account of methods would be incomplete without reference to the importance attached in professional courses to the educational value of discussion with students of their own progress. This was commonly regarded as a joint assessment between student and staff, an integral part of the process of learning, rather than judgement at a given point in time, though it was summarized for training records towards the end of the period. Frank discussion of their progress with students is encouraged by all training bodies and academic staff, though there were differences of view about whether or not students should see their reports, and some contrasts in practice. In one course, for example, the students not only saw and signed their own reports, but were invited to add their own comments; in another there was a rule against reports being shown to students.

Two students of professional courses wrote as follows:

Discussions were valuable with the supervisor because you felt trusted to know what was sent, and able to find out why if you did not know before the report was written as it was. . . . It also helped in going to the next placement as your next supervisor got a copy and you would both start off from the same place.

(Aged 31. One year course in Medical Social Work.)

They (i.e. reports) gave me greater insight into myself. They helped me to see the areas in which I was finding difficulty, and if these are recognized then they can be dealt with.

(Aged 25. First year of course leading to Certificate in Social Work.)

Summary and Implications.

There is considerable unanimity in the aims expressed by academic and field work staff for students from professional courses as compared with those from basic courses. At both stages certain methods are commonly used, but in the case of students from basic courses lack of clarity in purpose tends towards failure in offering experience related to other learning.

In professional training there is much agreement about and emphasis upon acquiring skill in individual relationships. Further study of the content and method of teaching would be needed to find out how well this serves the purpose of clients with varying practical and personal needs. Relatively little mention was made of the knowledge and skill involved in differentiating between the kinds of service needed.

Understanding of policy and administration was widely agreed to be important, but educational programmes for this purpose are relatively undeveloped or experimental.

TABLE IA: NUMBER OF FIELD WORK PLACEMENTS IN BASIC COURSES

Field work placements of at least four weeks made from courses in England, Scotland, Wales and Ireland (excluding *placements in* Ireland), during the year 1 October 1962 to 30 September 1963.

	Approxi-mate Length	Number of Courses	Number of Students Placed	Number of Place-ments
GRAND TOTAL FOR BASIC COURSES		54	935	1,228
UNIVERSITY Total	—	47	872	1,131
Degree	3 years	14	291	306
Post-graduate Diploma	1 year	16	241	350
Non-graduate Certificate or Diploma	2 years	17	340	475
UNIVERSITY OF LONDON		7	63	97
External Diploma in Social Studies { Full-time	2 years	1	6	10
Part time	3 years	4	32	50
Day release	2-5 years	1	3	5
Correspondence Course	2 years or more	1	22	32

NOTE.—All figures relate to the particular twelve month period. As courses vary in length and pattern these figures should not be read as referring to the number of placements arranged for students in each year of a course.

Field work placements of at least four weeks made from courses in England, Scotland, Wales and Ireland (excluding *placements in* Ireland), during the year 1 October 1962 to 30 September 1963.

	Approximate Length	Number of Courses	Number of Students Placed	Number of Placements
GRAND TOTAL FOR PROFESSIONAL COURSES	—	40	965	1,584
UNIVERSITY Total	—	19	356	631
Applied Social Studies (generic)	1 year	7	106	205
[1]Post-graduate (child care and probation)	17 to 18 months	4	109	151
Child care	1 year	3	66	98
Medical Social Work	1 year	1	9	25
Mental Health (psychiatric social work)	1 year	4	66	152
COLLEGES OF FURTHER EDUCATION or UNIVERSITY EXTRA-MURAL Total	—	13	273	450
Certificate in Social Work	2 years	7	155	242
Child Care (mature students)	1 year	1	20	26
Child Care	2 years	3	68	126
Probation (mature students)	1 year	1	17	37
Probation	2 years	1	13	19
OTHER ORGANIZATIONS Total	—	8	336	503
[2]Advisory Council for Probation and After Care	9 months to 1 year	4	206	295
C. of E. Council for Social Work and Moral Welfare	6 months / 2 years	1 / 1	39	62
Institute of Medical Social Workers	9 to 10 months	1	71	126
National Institute for Social Work Training (experienced staff)	1 year	1	20	20

[1] Graduates in subjects other than social sciences.

[2] Training of varying length and pattern for students of differing age and experience.

NOTE.—*All figures relate to the particular twelve month period. As courses vary in length and pattern these figures should be read as referring to the number of placements arranged for students in each year of a course.*

TABLE IIᴀ: PLACEMENT IN DIFFERENT TYPES OF AGENCY
BASIC AND PROFESSIONAL COURSES

PUBLIC SERVICES

Field work placements of at least four weeks (excluding residential) in England, Scotland and Wales during the year 1 October 1962 to 30 September 1963.

SOCIAL AGENCIES	BASIC AND PROFESSIONAL		BASIC		PROFESSIONAL	
	Number	%	Number	%	Number	%
Totals	1,879	100	614	100	1,265	100
CHILDREN'S DEPARTMENTS	473	25·2	152	24·8	321	25·4
MEDICAL SOCIAL WORK						
(1) Community Care	6 ⎫		4 ⎫		2 ⎫	
(2) General Practice	4 ⎬373	19·9	2 ⎬123	20·0	2 ⎬250	19·8
(3) Hospitals	363 ⎭		117 ⎭		246 ⎭	
MENTAL HEALTH SERVICES						
(1) Child Guidance Clinics	117 ⎫		17 ⎫		100 ⎫	
(2) Community Care	48 ⎬348	18·5	23 ⎬84	13·7	25 ⎬264	20·9
(3) Hospitals	183 ⎭		44 ⎭		139 ⎭	
PROBATION	593	31·6	175	28·5	418	33·0
PUBLIC HEALTH	23	1·1	18 ⎫		5 ⎫	
SCHOOL WELFARE	3	0·2	1 ⎬30	4·9	2 ⎬9	0·7
WELFARE DEPARTMENTS	13	0·7	11 ⎭		2 ⎭	
MISCELLANEOUS PLACEMENTS						
Administration, Local Government, etc.	11 ⎫		11 ⎫			
Community organization and development (New Towns, etc.)	13 ⎪		13 ⎪			
Education Departments	7 ⎬53	2·8	6 ⎬50	8·1	1 ⎫	
Employment Exchanges	12 ⎪		12 ⎪		⎬3	0·2
Housing Departments	4 ⎪		4 ⎪		⎪	
Rehabilitation or retraining	4 ⎪		2 ⎪		2 ⎭	
Schools (day)	2 ⎭		2 ⎭			

TABLE IIʙ

PLACEMENTS IN DIFFERENT TYPES OF AGENCY
BASIC AND PROFESSIONAL COURSES

VOLUNTARY SERVICES

Field work placements of at least four weeks (excluding residential) in England, Scotland and Wales during the year 1 October 1962 to 30 September 1963

SOCIAL AGENCIES	BASIC AND PROFESSIONAL		COURSES BASIC		PROFESSIONAL	
	No.	%	No.	%	No.	%
Totals	605	100	428	100	177	100
Adoption Societies	6	1·0	2	0·5	4	2·3
Care Committee (L.C.C.)	17	2·8	17	3·9		
Child Care	1	0·2			1	0·6
Citizen's Advice Bureau	20	3·3	20	4·7		
Community Organization or development	2	0·3	2	0·5		
Family Casework	371	61·3	247	57·7	124	70·0
Handicapped Persons	9	1·5	6	1·4	3	1·7
Invalid Children's Aid Association	34	5·6	26	6·0	8	4·5
Industrial (personnel and health)	19	3·2	19	4·5		
Moral Welfare	47	7·8	10	2·3	37	20·9
Old People's Welfare	3	0·5	3	0·7		
Prisoners (Discharged Aid)	2	0·3	2	0·5		
Settlements and Community Centres	69	11·4	69	16·1		
Youth Clubs and Recreation	5	0·8	5	1·2		

3

THE CHOICE OF FIELD WORK

THE difficulty of finding satisfactory opportunities of training in the field for students in professional courses was one of the main reasons for this Survey. This was also said to be true in the choice of suitable experience for students in basic courses. We now turn to consider how selections are made, on the one hand by academic staff and on the other by those responsible for social services who are asked to provide educational experience for students.

It has been seen that the main responsibility for the field work of students from both types of course falls upon the casework services. Certain difficulties therefore inevitably affect both types of course.

In the correspondence inquiry sent to academic staff arranging field work of any kind, four out of five were experiencing the following problems:

1. Shortage of staff in agencies otherwise suitable.

2. Keenness of competition between the staff of courses for a limited number of places for students.

3. The standard of service in nearby agencies.

Two other difficulties were experienced by half those who replied:

4. Lack of time to explore the position in agencies not so far asked to take students.

5. Lack of accommodation for staff and students in the agencies.

The means by which opportunities become known or are explored must be seen in the light of these facts. One tutor in Scotland described her desperation and ingenuity as 'plucking placements out of thin air.'

The different ways in which this general situation affects the staff of basic and professional courses will now be considered.

PART I

BASIC COURSES

Field work opportunities and the number of students

It is often said that students who might prove suitable for social work are rejected for initial courses. It seems important for this reason alone to discover how far opportunities for field work play a part in determining the number of students accepted.

The answer is that the acceptance of students is considerably affected by these opportunities, though not in any simple way. The staff of half the social study courses said that in the number admitted they were influenced by field work opportunities, sometimes because of general limitations and sometimes because they were looking for particular kinds of experience for their students.

Of the thirteen courses of which this was said to be true, five were in Scotland or Northern Ireland, and these comprised *all* the courses in these two areas. Special difficulties were reported from Scotland. Here there is an even more critical shortage of qualified social workers, particularly in the local authorities, where the total number was fourteen in the survey year, twelve of whom were employed in Children's Departments.

The number of students in the other eight English courses in which admissions were affected by field work, varied from eight to forty-six. The universities are widely scattered, five being north and three south of an east-west line running through Coventry. In five, it was stated that field work was only one of the influences in determining the number, the other being either the 'quota' for the department laid down by the university, or the time of the staff in tutoring and in visiting agencies. The following illustrations show a variety of considerations:

> The maximum number of students was set at fifteen originally because of the difficulty of obtaining suitable practical work experience for a larger number, *especially any introduction to case-work.** More recently, the number was also restricted by College policy. . . . It would be very difficult to find new pre-professional training possibilities in more specialized settings because we have not been allowed to expand numbers. We have always managed to obtain suitable experience in other fields than general family casework.
>
> (University: one year post-graduate course.)

* Italics added.

Another writer explains that she thinks it is important that at least one placement should give the opportunity 'to see a trained social worker in action' and that in at least one placement the students should be able 'to interview people in a social work situation under supervision'; this is one influence on the number of students accepted, though the College also sets limits.

(University: Two-year non-graduate, one year post-graduate courses.)

Methods of choice of the agencies

Knowledge about the agencies was received by academic staff in two main ways. The first of these is highly personal. The 'grape-vines' referred to by more than one correspondent seems a suitable description. The second is the use of certain central sources of information about the standard of the agencies.

Much reliance is placed upon cumulative knowledge of individual members of staff through correspondence and telephone conversations about students, through the students' own accounts, and from reports received on their work over the years. A few tutors visited the agencies at intervals; some only when difficulties occurred, others rarely. To these sources of knowledge are added personal encounters of all kinds, partly social, partly professional, building up information, particularly in the area of the course, about the standards of an agency and its staff. University staff, well known in their own communities, draw upon their contacts as magistrates, as members of committees and training boards, as participants in professional conferences, and on social occasions in common rooms, where the staff of different departments and professions share friendships and interests. For contacts at a distance it was acknowledged that reliance often had to be placed upon correspondence by letter and telephone even at the initial stage. Reference was made to the help of past students of particular courses, not only in receiving students themselves, but also in making suggestions about new opportunities.

Few of the staff regarded it as necessary or practical to ask for particular supervisors for their students, though some were personally well known to those who placed students locally. Some correspondents referred to the fact that, though they might in the first instance see the person who was 'administratively responsible' for the agency, this was likely to take place only at the beginning of a continuing arrangement.

This 'grape-vine' method may, with luck, lead to sound judgements but this must depend to a large extent upon the experience of individual members of the staff—their standing in the community, their particular interests and the number of years they have had for this capital investment. The legacy of individual experience is not easy to transmit. The very fact of its personal nature may encourage perseveration rather than fresh appraisal and exploration; this seems likely if only because of the value and security of relationships already established and the saving of precious time. Academic staff do not generally regard it as their responsibility to make a direct assessment of the quality of work of the agencies in which their students were placed. Only three, for example, had read any case records in the services in which their students were placed.

A number referred to the help they received from those who could assess agencies for training. One of these sources is the list of voluntary casework agencies drawn up as a result of their appraisal by the Joint Committee on Family Casework Training. Another is the headquarters staff or regional inspectorate of certain services. A third is the professional organizations, guided by members who hold their qualification.

The only example of a combined attempt to appraise agencies for the training of students from basic courses is that undertaken by the Joint Committee on Family Casework Training. This Committee, started in 1941, has drawn up certain standards relating to the qualifications of the supervisor, the casework undertaken and the records kept. Representatives of the Committee visit the organization, discuss their work with the staff and read case records. 'Approved' agencies are included on a special list and this inclusion has been held to entitle them to fees. The work of the Committee has been carried out under difficulties, and different views were expressed in the Survey about its effectiveness. The principle of such an assessment, and its use by the staff of a variety of courses is of obvious importance.

Difficulties experienced by staff in placing students

It has been seen that the main blocks take place on the roads that lead to casework agencies. This early experience of casework is regarded by some academic staff as crucial to the future professional progress of the students; the choice of agency then seemed to them to be as important for students from basic courses as it was for those at the later stage of their training, though the criteria were different. Some staff were doubtful about the suitability of the teaching given in certain agencies where methods were more geared to professional students, and this was restricting their choice.

Competition for places, particularly during vacation periods, was

D

felt to be specially serious in certain areas, as the following examples will show:

> In areas where applied social studies courses have been developed many of the casework agencies pledge their resources in these courses as much as a year in advance, and also tend to commit vacancies they may have for pre-professional students in advance on a block basis. Thus, although there is a convention that family casework vacancies for the June and September period should not be committed until the 1st February, for other times in the year it is often necessary to ask for a placement at least nine months before it is wanted. This makes nonsense of planning because in the interval the student's development may indicate a different form of training. Because it is impossible to get any worthwhile casework placement at short notice, one is generally forced to put the student in a wrong agency.
>
> (University: non-graduate two-year course.)

> In one area, we were told, placements for casework experience have become 'particularly desperate' and may have reached 'saturation point'. This was illustrated by the difficulty in getting any placement at all for a late entrant. A search was made by telephone in about twenty agencies from which the kind of reply received was that they had had 'so many students that they simply couldn't face another at the moment' and they seemed, as it was graphically put, 'squeezed and exhausted'.
>
> (Degree, non-graduate two-year and post-graduate one-year courses.)

Exploring new opportunities

It has been said that half those who replied referred to the lack of time of the academic staff to explore new possibilities of valuable experience. Heart-felt wishes were expressed for a wider range of choice. One member of staff wrote that the lack of time of the staff to visit agencies and discuss the needs of their students was probably the greatest difficulty in expanding field work; another, responsible for many students, said she thought there were numbers of agencies and individuals in the country where students could be supervised if they could only be discovered and helped in the early stages. The claims of a heavy teaching programme or of research had to be weighed against the time needed for this sort of exploration and help. However, a number were doubtful whether the search for, and selection of agencies would be useful unless it were done by those who were able to judge their suitability for the students of a particular course.

The possibility of giving help to the staff of agencies who might feel diffident about their ability to supervise students raises important questions which will be discussed later. Here it should be noted that academic staff particularly welcomed special programmes of teaching arranged for groups of students in relation to their practical work, and this influenced their choice of agencies, for example, settlements and certain casework agencies.

Accommodation and financial considerations

The lack of adequate physical accommodation proved to have limited the opportunities for no less than half those who replied. Reference is made to such chronic over-crowding in certain agencies that 'there is no space for another chair for a student and no privacy'. In some instances space and equipment is the only reason why a good supervisor cannot accept one or more than one student. In Scotland lack of office accommodation has severely limited the number of students.

It has been difficult to estimate to what extent financial considerations influence the choice of agencies. The academic staff were asked a specific question about fees paid to agencies. In only four courses was this mentioned as a difficulty and in two of these it was regarded as relatively unimportant. Since this date there has, however, been discussion about fees[1] between a number of voluntary organizations concerned with training and this is continuing at the time of publication.

The influence of the financial circumstances of students is often partly concealed by a number of other facts. One of these is the importance attached to the student's own choice of area and type of agency for his field work. Motives of economy as well as other factors are involved here. Only a sixth of the staff who replied regarded the financial circumstances of students as important in carrying out their plans, but half found that their choice of placements was affected in a relatively unimportant way, by such difficulties as the authorization by grant-aiding authorities of claims for travelling and other expenses incurred by students during their field work. Part of the problem was the variety of the financial circumstances of individual students. Here, for example, is the statement of a member of staff with experience of a large number of students:

All grant-aiding authorities should pay adequate extra grants to

[1] Standing Conference of Councils of Social Service, National Council of Social Service, *Memorandum prepared by representatives of seven national voluntary organizations and six councils of social service regarding appropriate fees to be charged for Certificate in Social Work students by those voluntary casework agencies who provide long term tractical work placements*, 1964.

cover field work expenses. It seems wrong that generous statutory or voluntary agencies should be asked to pay fares when students are accompanying workers in order to increase their own knowledge, or to provide board and lodging where students are not temporary members of the staff, but are in the agency for their own education.

The source from which students receive their grants affects the choice of area for individuals. If the family is paying, means are generally much more limited. Residential placements may be chosen for this reason. If they receive local authority grants these tend to be skimpy and the student may find it difficult to manage.

(Degree, post-graduate one year and non-graduate two year courses.)

Students' own choices

Students are generally encouraged in the first instance to express their preference for the type of field work and the area in which it is to be undertaken, partly because this is seen as a good principle in adult education, partly with a view to economy. One head of a department who wondered why her colleagues became so exercised about the placement of their students during the early stages of their training, and whose students spent one period of their field work as 'student employees' in various commercial establishments, thought that their initiative was important in learning 'to stand on their own feet'. 'The students are not drafted, they are helped . . . they generally choose wisely . . . they help each other'. The wisdom of the choice is carefully considered by staff and student before it is authorized by the university, and the staff decision does not necessarily coincide with the student's request.

Sometimes it was clear to the staff that the student's choice was mainly determined by economy—their need, as it was put, 'to live in their homes or cheap places'. Sometimes their choice was based upon whether they could be near relatives or friends, and it was recognized as important for some students not to feel isolated.

The students themselves evidently think it important that they should be consulted. In the inquiry addressed by the committee of the Association of Social Work and Social Study Students to their members the first question ran 'Were your wishes taken into account regarding the choice of area and agency?' Three quarters of 104 undertaking block periods of field work *were* consulted by their tutors about the area to which they went. Of this number, half, not living at home during the term, were with their families while they did practical work;

just under a third went into 'new' lodgings, and the rest stayed in their term-time residence whether at home or in lodgings. It is not known how far questions of economy dictated the choice for the students who went to live at home during their periods of field work, but it seems likely to have been an important factor.

The influence of students' preferences may extend the range of the agencies chosen, but it must be difficult for students with their limited experience to compare opportunities. It must also be difficult for the staff to learn enough about the widely scattered agencies suggested by students to be sure that the decision is the best one. Indeed, there was evidence of this from the field, and the problem was acknowledged by one member of the academic staff who referred to the need to have time to explore:

> New placements ought to be found and cherished, but there is no time. Admittedly, it is at present haphazard . . . students give me ideas . . . someone is met on holiday somewhere.

Opinions of the staff of social agencies

Chapter 2 has already referred to the welcome given to students by the staff of agencies and this for the most part applied, in spite of the special difficulties, to those who were young or inexperienced as well as to others. A number of senior staff, as well as those who actually supervised these students, spoke of the benefits that they brought to the agency in terms of enjoyment, interest, encouragement and challenge. About two thirds of the senior staff personally consulted—such as children's officers, senior medical social workers, organizing secretaries of voluntary agencies—described a number of difficulties, but made light of them compared with their interest in taking a share in the training of future social workers; about a fifth described very considerable problems. Few seemed to have doubts about continuing to receive students. About three-fifths of the agencies consulted were receiving students both from basic and from professional courses.

Part of the incentive towards this welcoming attitude to students from basic courses was the hope of attracting qualified candidates to their particular service in the future. Another influence was personal loyalty to the staff of certain courses in which a valued partnership had grown up through the years. There was often a combination of these motives in accepting a proportion of degree and certificate students from local courses. The sorting out of requests received at different times of year, sometimes with little notice, becomes a very complicated matter, particularly because of the number of different courses from which students come, the varied length and pattern of training, and seasonal pressures. Nearly half the agencies taking both types of students received them from five or more training departments and nearly a third provided field work for students of five or more different types of course. One agency received students from eleven different courses and two others from as many as nine.

The difficulty of sorting out priorities in the midst of this multitude of requests was well illustrated by a Principal Probation Officer and a Children's Officer:

Probation Service

Although 'committed' to probation course students, whether from generic or specific courses and stating on behalf of his service, 'we *must* interest uncommitted students', this Principal Probation Officer feels an obligation to social work generally and a great concern for 'the undergraduate stage'. In one year he was only able to take 5 out of 22 applications from basic course students. In this choice preference was given to those who lived in the area, partly because of longstanding partnership with the staff of a particular course. A further influence on the acceptance of local basic course students was that these students would be more likely to become recruits to their particular agency because they lived nearby. When at the basic course stage these students came to them he made a point of keeping in touch with them and hoped for an application for a post 'several years ahead'. The Committee was said to be carried along in their support of training because 'what you put in you are likely to get out', and 'the greatest incentive is the end result'.

(County Probation Service. Number of officers: 60. Number of staff supervising students: 29. Students are also received from kindred types of training, e.g. for residential staff.)

Children's Department

The Children's Officer says she is most anxious to take a full share in the training of students, but although she receives basic course students from four different educational bodies, she would prefer to concentrate on those who come from professional courses for child care officers and, in fact, would favour a special training centre for these particular students. At the same time, she had only positive statements to make about the effect of students in general upon the work of a busy department. 'It is always useful to have students in that it brings existing staff into touch with

new thought.' She went on to say that constant new thinking was vital and 'if we have a daft system we had better change it!'
(County Children's Department. Number of child care officers: 10. Number supervising students: 3.)

Complexity of motives is also illustrated when particular problems are described. Many of these difficulties relate to confusion about purposes, which has been considered in the last chapter and anticipate the methods of communication between courses and agencies to be discussed in the next. However, even in the initial acceptance of students there are problems not only of priority, but other difficulties, of which the following appear to be the most important:

1. *Staff shortage*
Most of the agencies used for field work, some with expanding responsibilities, were suffering from unfilled vacancies and from frequent changes of staff.

2. *Staff establishment*
In the view of senior staff, closely connected with the overall staff shortage is the lack of recognition on the part of some training bodies and employers of the time needed by staff for students.

3. *Conflict between responsibility for their own junior or newly appointed staff, and students*
This particular problem was mentioned by local authorities concerned about the supervision of their unqualified staff and by certain voluntary organizations where more basic course students might otherwise have been welcomed. For example:

> *Voluntary organization*
> Here it was thought that basic course students should only occasionally be received, partly because of the C.A.B. prior obligation to their own staff and partly because some of their cases were thought to be unsuitable for students from basic courses. The length of time for students had, therefore, become limited to two weeks and it was thought that there must be 'long gaps in between'.
> (*Citizens Advice Bureau*. Regular staff: 1. Voluntary workers: 24. Trainees: 2.)

4. *Obligations to clients*
It is of interest to notice that, apart from the conflict involved in the time given to students, the question of the suitability of students from

basic courses from the point of view of clients was seldom mentioned. This is probably because, for the most part, they were regarded as 'observers' at this stage in their training. Nevertheless, reference was made by certain agencies (and is illustrated in the last example) to the fact that only certain kinds of cases were 'suitable' for students at early stages in their experience. Sometimes the student's own choice, leading to a placement near his home or for other practical reasons, but not suitable from the standpoint of the work of the agency, caused difficulties partly because of local connection and led to reluctance to take another student, but this seemed rare.

Certain definite limitations are placed upon the experience which can be offered to any students by the Ministry of Labour and the National Assistance Board because of their regulations about the confidential nature of records and personal contact with clients. Students are only allowed to listen to staff interviews, and are sometimes only shewn 'dummy' case records. The criteria by which these particular public services were differentiated from others were not easy to discover. Observance of confidence is a cherished principle in all training for social work. There is wide acceptance in public and private social services that it is proper for responsible students under competent supervision to be brought within the closed circuit of privileged communication. In the National Health Service, for example, where medical confidence is also involved, supervised students are trusted within proper limits; in the probation service, where legal issues are involved, safeguards are established and accepted.

Summary: choice of field work for students from basic courses

Large numbers of students from basic courses are placed in the same casework agencies as those from professional courses with resulting competition. Their placement is not with consistency based upon first-hand knowledge of what the agencies have to offer. Increased competition is setting severe limits upon choice. Academic staff are anxious for more opportunities. There is widespread interest in these students in the agencies, partly based upon the hope of recruitment. In their decisions about the acceptance of students, agency staff are bewildered by a variety of applications, conflicting loyalties and erratic timing. In spite of much interest and goodwill, the lines are often crossed in such a way as to frustrate the purposes of callers at both ends, anxious in the interests of students to hear and to understand one another.

PART II

PROFESSIONAL COURSES

There are important differences between the patterns of professional courses, but certain common characteristics distinguish the problems of choice of field training from those that have so far been discussed. Almost all these students are training for casework, and this is the touchstone of their learning, although they may also undertake other types of field work for short periods. The fact that casework is their ultimate concern is recognized from the outset both by the staff of the agencies and of the courses, and there is obviously better mutual understanding of the purpose of the exercise, and more engagement of both parties in its pursuit.

The differences between professional courses are however likely to have important implications for the agencies. There are twelve different patterns of professional training, half requiring students to have completed certain basic courses and half making no such condition, but designed from the start as a sequence leading to professional qualification. Even within this general scheme, there are important modifications made for students of different ages and experience. A further condition is that a proportion of these courses depend upon local field work because of a 'concurrent' pattern of training, whereas others often send their students to a distance for periods of full-time practice.

Academic staff of professional courses attach immense importance to learning and teaching in the field. One head of a university department said 'The supervisors are just as much—indeed *more* a part of the educational process than we are'.

Influence of field work opportunities on the number of students
The staff of half the basic courses stated that the intake of their students was to some extent determined by field work opportunities; this compares with about four fifths of the professional courses (28 out of 33). In nearly a third it is these opportunities *alone* which determine the exact upper limit for the intake of students. Six out of seven of the universities, however, also have other reasons for setting this limit. The number of academic staff, determined by university policy, affects the time available for the development of field training.

The high proportion of professional courses in which the exact intake of students is limited by field work opportunities lends particular interest to exceptions, for which there seemed four different reasons:

(1) long established professional relationships between college and services based initially on psychiatric social work; (2) willingness to scatter students for block periods at a distance from their courses, with special tutorial arrangements in regions; (3) the choice of particular voluntary services which students from a certain college are likely to enter; (4) success in developing sufficient support for local field work training. An interesting example of the fourth situation was an area in which, within a period of about five years, with the help of student units, qualified supervisors had been found for the students of two new professional courses. Here there had been energetic promotion of interest and partnership for which the staff of a university and college of further education had worked closely together, and where special efforts had been made to interest the chief officers of local services. The limitation of students in the university was said at this stage to depend upon the shortage of *academic* staff; on this account, there might even be some wastage of carefully fostered field work opportunities. There were examples in other areas of this expansion, but each gain seemed to be overtaken by a more rapid increase of students.

Views of academic staff about the choice of field work

The main difference from the basic courses in the decisions made at the professional stage is the great importance attached by academic staff to the choice of the individual supervisor, and to the principle that this should be a matter of agreement between them and the staff responsible for the agency. Initially interviews are held with senior staff in charge, but as time goes on the arrangement tends to be regarded as a general sanction for those who supervise to undertake all the responsibilities of the partnership.

The staff of these courses also make use of central sources of information, but they too rely to a considerable extent upon cumulative knowledge from a variety of sources. In Scotland it was stated that 'except where student units exist, choice of tutors is always based on personal knowledge of the individual and the agency. This knowledge is gathered by the 'grapevine' system. Assuming certain basic standards in an agency, the personal qualities of the supervisor determines the choice'. The fact that many of the students are placed with local agencies provides more opportunities for reliable information. Not all those with whom we discussed the initial stages of selection were satisfied, however, that they had sufficient facts upon which to base their own inquiries, as the following illustration shows:

The staff said that it was difficult for new tutors in a new course to get to know people in the agencies. They did this by visiting and by 'the grape-vine'. The visit is 'a more methodical way', 'the grape-vine very chancy'. The tutor would like to have a public list of agencies and work through it steadily; she thinks the present way of getting to know about supervisors is wasteful and inefficient; there are people who could be supervisors and are being missed, but it needs time to look for them.

(College of Further Education. Certificate in Social Work Course.)

Some of those who consulted regional inspectors of public services were not always satisfied that they were able to appraise services from the standpoint of training.

Central councils organizing training for certain services have, each in their own field, sources of information about staff and certain priorities upon which they can rely for placements in their own service. This does not imply that they are necessarily exclusive about the use of 'their' service, or that they are unaffected by pressures. Again, a professional organization providing training has sources of information and goodwill of a special nature among its members, often consisting of past students.

When the final choice of supervisor rests with the staff of courses there is a different relationship with those who are in charge of agencies, as we shall see when we turn to their side of the story. Delicate problems of diplomacy are involved. Criteria of choice may be difficult as the following illustration shows:

The academic staff member in charge of a course in applied social studies said that the first criterion of choice was the professional qualification of the field work staff, but added 'this does not take you very far' (in terms of opportunities in this area). It should be made clear to the agencies in the first instance that the selection of supervisors without professional qualifications is an exception. If those without qualifications are chosen it is important that they should have been doing a job for some time and 'know what it is about'. The person who is chosen must be 'encouraging and appreciative', 'not too anxious and not trying to solve their own problems'. They must be able to communicate, to 'know what they are doing and why'.

(University. Course in Applied Social Studies.)

While it is the general view that supervisors should hold professional qualification, it was accepted by the majority of staff that to limit the choice of agencies from this standpoint alone would, in the early development of courses, make exapnsion of training impossible. Some had found very gifted supervisors among those with no professional qualifications for social work. Two main methods of getting over this hurdle have been adopted. The first of these is to appoint a member of staff in certain agencies for the supervision of a group of students; the other to devise means of preparing staff for the work of supervision and of supporting them while they are undertaking it. In the twelve professional courses in which interviews were held, seven were dependent upon units; in three others, discussion was going forward about their establishment. (See Chapter 5, p. 85.)

The second approach to the problem, that of helping to prepare and to support the field work staff concerned with students, is central to the interests of this Survey and is considered in the next chapter. It is important in the choice of field work because seminars organized for those who are supervising or who might undertake this responsibility in the future have proved to be one of the most valuable means of discovering individuals who have educational ability. This is well illustrated in the following account:

> Those in charge of this course said that there must be sufficient time for supervisors to 'absorb new knowledge and make use of it' before they are able to pass it on to students. 'They must digest it in order to be simple about it.' This capacity is not necessarily related to their own training, though the staff thought that all supervisors should have professional qualifications; essential and no less important are personal maturity and skill. A period of preparation is necessary.

In this course difficulty was experienced in finding enough places regarded as suitable and the reasons for this are pertinent:

1. Appointment of the best supervisors to academic posts of teaching or research.

2. Exhaustion of field work staff from too heavy a programme of casework and supervision.

3. Responsibility for students considered by administrative staff to be too extravagant in terms of staff time.

The outcome of these difficulties was the establishment of a student unit.

(Certificate in Social Work Course.)

So much stress is laid upon the choice of individual supervisors that the standard of the whole service sometimes appears to be of less concern. The qualifications for supervision of individual members of the staff occasionally led to the placement of a student in an agency not otherwise approved. In some areas, however, the nearest and most appropriate agencies were *not* used for training because of what was regarded as an unprogressive department, or the absence, shortage, or frequent changes of qualified staff. The impact and combination of these and other problems is crucial if, because of the concurrent pattern of the course (i.e. weekly field work), students must be placed within easy travelling distance.

Accommodation and financial considerations

About two thirds of those who replied about particular difficulties instanced problems of accommodation. Examples were given of congested offices which made it impossible to accept a student, and of agencies in which more students could have worked with one skilled supervisor if space had been available. The expense of overnight lodgings or of mileage allowances for students in areas where suitable experience can only be gained by the use of cars have sometimes limited the choice of field work. Agencies have been generous in covering travelling expenses of student casework where these are not met from public training funds, but anomalies sometimes caused irritation.

Some difficulties in the choice of agencies would clearly be eased, but not solved, if there were more knowledge available about agencies and the qualifications of staff. An immense amount of time is spent by the staff of both prospective and established courses combing the ground in search of promising field work for their students. The staff take the view that personal discussion is essential for mutual understanding about the courses and the particular needs of their students, partly because they want to make a personal appraisal of the agency for training and partly because introductions may be the beginning of partnership. Important as all these purposes may be, a number of such visits may be abortive, and the use of time by skilled staff must be seen as a question of central concern in future developments.

This review of the choice of field work for students from professional courses suggests many problems, but the academic staff recognize encouraging signs. The following note was offered by a university lecturer of long experience:

> I should like to comment on the greatly increased interest in student training shown nowadays in all social agencies. This was most noticeable at the recent meetings we called at the university of the heads of all social agencies we might wish to use. There was (full) attendance and real keenness.

Opinions of the staff of social agencies

In professional courses the welcome extended to students took on a special significance. This was undoubtedly partly due to the regard for the agency and its staff implied in being selected for training. For example:

> (these students are) a compliment to the agency . . . in a sense it is like a teaching hospital . . . we gain. To have students is a two-way thing—it attracts and holds staff . . . senior staff who would think twice about coming and staying without students.
>
> (County Children's Department. Students received from several professional courses.)

This sense of privilege and participation seemed for the senior staff to outweigh the considerable pressure resulting from the time expected of their supervisors in direct work with students and the meetings they were expected to attend.

Qualifications of Supervisors

The qualifications of supervisors are of central importance, not only in their own right, but because their own experience in training is likely to affect the views they hold. The returns received on 112 supervisors of professional course students in England showed that 69 per cent had themselves received professional training, while 13 per cent had only basic qualifications. The remainder had some other type of academic or professional qualification, or, in a few cases, none at all. A number had attended special short courses or conferences on supervision in addition to the regular seminars involved in the training of their students. In the Scottish survey similar proportions were found in the qualifications of 51 supervisors of students in basic and professional courses.

The staff who supervised students from professional courses had two chief incentives. One was their interest in training students for the service in which they themselves were employed; the other their close identification with a neighbouring course from which students came for concurrent field work. The majority of students who were intending to enter the service in which they were training came for block periods; and it was, therefore, difficult to distinguish the two motives. It was however interesting to find expressions of relief and enthusiasm from a few probation officers who could reconcile these two incentives when they began to receive probation students from a nearby course with which they could become closely identified. We were told by the staff responsible nationally for placing probation students that other probations officers preferred those who could concentrate entirely on the service rather than taking students for concurrent field work. In the Survey areas great appreciation was expressed both by probation officers and other social workers of the encouragement they received from meeting with other supervisors in close consultation with the staff of courses from which the students came.

Why did concurrent field work hold such attractions? It seems clear, that the main influence at work is the much closer partnership established between the staff of the agencies and the courses. The nature of this partnership will be considered in the next chapter. It is important in this context because of the effect it appears to have upon the spread of good opportunities for professional training and upon priorities in the acceptance of students.

SUMMARY AND IMPLICATIONS

Students from basic and professional courses compete for supervised experience in casework services. In most professional courses the exact number of students admitted is crucially affected by opportunities for field training. Here, in contrast to basic courses, the choice of individual supervisor is the main consideration.

In the choice of placements central sources of information are used, but in both courses much reliance is placed upon individual enquiry, liable in basic courses to be subject to chance and in professional courses very time-consuming. Office accommodation and travelling distance limits placements.

Agencies have difficulty in using consistent criteria for selection; the two main influences appear to be the attraction of local courses offering close partnership and concern for the needs of their own service.

There are examples of notable expansion achieved by providing opportunities for study and consultation to local social workers.

More distinction appears to be needed between the claims on agencies of students from basic and professional courses; more comprehensive knowledge about field work resources for both; and more consultation between agencies, courses and training councils in considering priorities.

4

PARTNERSHIP IN TRAINING

Two aspects of communication are involved in the field work of students, whether it be regarded mainly as observation, or as acquiring professional skill. One is the function of this experience in the course as a whole; the other, the progress and assessment of individual students. Academic staff, field work supervisors and the students themselves must all be concerned with ways in which mutual understanding affects learning and teaching. Integration in learning depends to a large extent upon the initiative, receptiveness and discernment of the students themselves; nevertheless, if they are to be encouraged to learn co-herently from study and practice the staff responsible need to be clear with one another about purposes and methods. We may legitimately ask, therefore, how this understanding on both sides is initiated and fostered.

It has already been found that the responsibilities of field work supervisors are seen differently by the academic staff of basic and professional courses. The ways in which these differences work out in practice will now be considered.

PART I

BASIC COURSES

The increase of professional courses and students has added problems of competition to the existing difficulties of communication between academic staff and social workers receiving students from basic courses. Students cannot so easily be placed nearby, or with staff known through past contacts. Some plans are inevitably dictated by expediency. If the outcome is regarded by some as reasonably satisfactory this is probably due to the evident interest and goodwill on both sides, and on occasion to a 'little bit of luck'. One experienced member of staff, wondering whether she was too optimistic, said, 'It is very rare for practical work to go wrong . . . most students enjoy it and get a lot from it'. Many of the staff however were troubled about present conditions and future developments. The whole subject has been a matter of concern and deliberation in the Joint University Council for Social and Public Administration.

There are contrasting views held by senior academic staff about the extent to which university teachers should be concerned with field work. One professor in charge of a department including both basic and professional courses acknowledged that those who supervised students in the field should have help in the study of their methods, but thought that this should be the business of 'institutes of social work training' rather than of universities. At the other extreme, there were examples of universities in which field work was thought to be so important in relation to study that academic staff supervised students in the agency. One motive for this arrangement was illustrated in the tutor's comment, 'The university department (in this way) has a direct and detailed knowledge of the student's capacity and achievement in this field.'

Academic staff in charge of basic courses assumed that the main responsibility for helping the student to relate practice and study rested with their university tutors, but it was generally accepted that some degree of educational guidance must be given by their supervisors. Questions about communication seemed to them to be cogent.

Methods of academic staff

Much reliance is placed upon correspondence by letter and telephone. Within an area, there may be considerable discussion between the tutors of some courses and individual supervisors, but agencies are seldom visited in connection with the placement of students. Over half the staff said that they did not visit at all, and, with the exception of one tutor who visited all her students, the rest did so only 'sometimes' or 'seldom'. In the Scottish report it was said that tutors, already overloaded, tended to rely upon 'contact if anything goes badly wrong', and added that supervisors felt that they were expected to 'manage on their own'. This seems broadly characteristic of the position elsewhere.

The usual method is for correspondence going from the university to the agency to refer briefly to the course that the student is taking and the purpose of this particular experience, giving certain particulars about the student. Requests are almost always made for reports from the agency, and headings for the content of these reports are often suggested.

For their knowledge of what the agency provides, academic staff

E

place considerable reliance upon the student's own account of his experience and upon the report on his work. The majority of the staff replying to a question about whether they had sufficient knowledge of what the agencies offered, were satisfied in this respect, but about a third replied that this was only true 'sometimes', and one tutor said that she was never well enough informed about the agency from the standpoint of training. A few tutors are able to draw upon their own recent experience in the field, but this is exceptional.

One means of coming to a clearer understanding on both sides is by meetings of supervisors. The wide scatter of students obviously sets limits to attendance. In nearly half the courses, however, supervisors were annually invited to the university. Some of these meetings are used to explain the nature of different courses about which the agency staff said they had insufficient knowledge when requests were received in writing. Others are of a social character, a gesture of appreciation rather than a means of mutual exchange about the content and method of training. There were signs that the need for meetings of this kind were becoming recognized, as the following illustration shows:

> I have a social gathering with a speaker for all who take students. . . . I have started a discussion group of supervisors who have taken second term students and hope that this may develop into a sort of Basic Course Supervisor's Working Party. So little is written about supervision outside professional courses that there is considerable vagueness about aims and expectations.
> (University: non-graduate two year and post-graduate one year course.)

The present position was regarded as unsatisfactory by nearly half the academic staff. Those who did not seek for change tended to regard the tutors as entirely responsible for the educational aspects of field work. Practical experience, according to this view, was likely to help the student to discover something of interest to his studies, but was not seen as an opportunity for the social worker to teach 'live' from his experience. Sometimes there seemed an almost deliberate casualness about consultation with those responsible for supervision—'I know the secretaries (of a voluntary organization) . . . I pop in and see them when I am in X . . . I get a feed back from the students'.

Difficulties described by academic staff

Academic staff who were dissatisfied with present methods of communication referred to the difficulty of conveying knowledge about different courses to those in the field; to the need for reciprocal understanding of the two aspects of learning, and to certain problems relating to individual students.

These difficulties are illustrated in the following comments:

> The major difficulty in communication is to get it over to supervisors that degree students are very different from 'certificate' students. They are younger—more academic in ways of thinking about social problems, and intelligent, taught to think critically and to question assumptions, and they are relatively inexperienced and at the stage of placement have very little direct teaching about social services and will therefore need both to observe and to be told a good deal before they can undertake any work on their own, though if there are jobs they can do these are very greatly appreciated by the students.
>
> (University: degree course.)

> There should be far more contact between academic and agency staff, but this is not possible at the present, owing to lack of personnel at the university. Very rarely is an agency visited purely to establish a personal contact concerning a student at the pre-professional stage of learning.
>
> (University: degree; one year post-graduate and
> two year non-graduate course.)

> More frequent meetings (are needed), between supervisors and staff of courses, more informal and continuous contacts, more opportunity for staff of courses to spend some time in various agencies, not merely to pay rather inspectorial visits before or when the students are attached.
>
> (University: one year post-graduate course.)

One tutor thought that if sufficient staff were available three meetings should be held with a supervisor of a student placed for four weeks or more—one before, one during, and one after placement. A very experienced practical work tutor, supporting the need for more discussion with supervisors, thought that visits to the agency while the student was there made for an artificial triangular situation and detracted from the supervisor's responsibility.

Exchanges about individual students reflect the degree of confidence between staff and their respect for students. There was concern on the part of some of the academic staff about the kinds of information which should be shared. Some tutors thought it right that personal facts, such as family affairs or tendency to anxiety, if these had a direct bearing upon their work, should be passed on only with the student's consent.

Some made a distinction between giving personal information and suggesting to the agency what they called 'areas of difficulty'. Examples were occasionally given of serious problems which it was thought could have been avoided by better understanding on both sides. In one of these the choice of casework with psychiatric patients had activated personal difficulties; in another, a 'eulogistic report' on a student from an agency was said to have by-passed problems which were recognized, but not passed on, and which led to discontinued training.

Reports from agencies on students

Most tutors regard reports on the field work of students as important in the estimate of their capabilities, qualified by such knowledge as they have of conditions in the agencies. The universities vary in the weight they attach to these reports in the award of certificates. Our information about this was incomplete. We were told that in many of the courses practical work reports were not crucial for academic qualification. Basic courses are no longer regarded as qualifying for social work, and this was said to affect the importance attached to field work reports. Instances were however given of the deferment of certificate award on account of unsatisfactory reports and of students encouraged to withdraw from courses for the same reason. For students applying for professional training the standard of their field work reports from basic courses, forming part of their whole record, may be of importance to their future careers. Aims, opportunities and standards seem, therefore, to call for careful joint consideration and it is difficult to see how this can be achieved by correspondence.

The majority of the academic staff thought it desirable that their reports should be discussed by supervisors with students. It is clear that they could not rely on such discussions taking place (see Chapter 2, p. 32). It seemed for the most part to be regarded as a function of the tutor to make educational use of the reports with the students. For tutors not closely in touch with the staff of the agency discussion of reports with students must often be a very difficult exercise.

The majority seemed satisfied that most of the reports gave an adequate account of the student's experience and the use he made of it. There was some indication that they failed to show clearly whether students had understood the *organization* of the service in which they worked. This theme recurs in other parts of the Survey.

Views of field work staff

It is evident from the emphatic opinions frequently expressed by social workers that there is insufficient exchange with the academic staff both about the content of courses and about students. A few of the supervisors are not concerned about this exchange, but the large majority are, and many of them find it difficult to get to know enough about the courses and how the experience they offer contributes towards the student's progress. Some of those who themselves trained in similar courses said that they had to rely upon their own past experience, but that they knew little or nothing of recent developments except from the student after his arrival. Understandably, there was much more interchange with local courses, though even so there were surprising exceptions.

There was sufficient variety of practice in communication to provide illuminating comparisons. Much appreciation was expressed when one or two tutors came from a distance to the agency; even one such discussion could apparently produce a completely changed outlook towards a particular course and its students. These descriptions showed that the failure to create any sense of partnership was felt as much, perhaps even more, than the lack of information. This attitude was illustrated in the following comments:

> The supervisor spoke with great appreciation of close contacts with local courses and of a tutor who regularly visited from a distance. She wondered whether there was much value in merely receiving syllabuses of what students were taught. She would like to continue receiving students through the tutor who visited regularly because 'we've got a contact and know where we are'. She added 'on the whole, we just don't know what they are doing . . . generally speaking, we get the feeling that they (the students) are not in their courses learning anything of relevance to what they do here.'
>
> (Family casework agency. Students received from seven basic courses.)

> We have so many students at so many different stages. Sometimes the universities do not give you a notion of what they want . . . with the professional courses you know what you are talking about' (but with these others) . . . no one ever comes near you.
>
> (Children's Department. Students received from a variety of basic and local professional courses.)

> There is only contact with the local tutor. The supervisor has never seen a tutor in the office from any other university and

sums up this situation 'tutors are egg-bound in their university!'
(Family casework agency. Students received from
three basic courses.)

Over the years we have done a great deal of training, but we have
always felt out on a limb and not in the swim . . . we have had a
very high proportion of professionally qualified staff and they feel
that the sort of training they can really give is at the casework
level and they do not take too kindly to the social science level.
(Children's Department. Students received from a large
variety of basic and two distant professional courses.)

Social work staff expressed considerable dissatisfaction also about
the way in which individual students were prepared for field work,
the inadequate information they received about certain students and
the part that their assessment of the student's progress played in the
appraisal of his achievement. An interesting difference emerged here
between the views expressed in our interviews in the areas in which
there were local basic and professional courses, and in the correspondence inquiry sent to counties within which there were no courses
of either kind. The staff of 'distant' agencies seemed, perhaps inevitably,
to settle for what they received, and offered much less criticism. This
and other evidence suggests that experience of partnership creates a
different point of view about the value of consultation. There were
however a few comments from the more distant counties that they
thought the position unsatisfactory and that a remedy should be
found:

Difficulties of distance rather than goodwill mean that communication is largely by letter. This is not really good enough on
either side.
(County Children's Department. Students received
from three basic courses.)

Stress was laid throughout on the need for personal discussions,
but social workers were also dissatisfied with some of the written
information, the timing of certain reports, the absence of any subsequent
news about the student in whom they were interested and which would
enable them to assess the part that they had played in training.
This represents how it seemed to some of the agency staff:

We are always a bit in the dark as to how students have been
prepared . . . some come with quite unreal expectations . . . some
expect to do what they call 'deep casework' . . . our only contact

is a bit of paper that arrives before the student comes (she then referred to the invaluable discussion she had with some tutors).

It would be helpful if the whole thing became more alive said another member of the staff of this agency.

(Voluntary family casework. Students received from a variety of basic and professional courses.)

More drastic criticisms were sometimes made:

The probation officer compared her 'complete ignorance' about certain of the students who came for their block placements with the careful introduction from the local professional course. Not only were there gaps in information about the first group, but the correspondence was sometimes 'sloppy and careless' and she instanced a promised letter which never came.

(Probation officer. Supervised students from a variety of basic courses and one from a local professional course.)

In the same area a probation officer compared two basic courses. From one she had *no* information until the tutor visited; from another she had 'a good pen picture' from the tutor, was sent a photograph, was told a little about the student's home background and the 'areas' of difficulty she might have.

Field workers as well as academic staff gave occasional examples of serious consequences of failure to consult. Two students caused anxiety to social workers because of severe depression, and one with acute asthma was sent to a very unsuitable area. An experienced supervisor, giving one such example, said that she had never seen a university tutor from outside the area and added that she often wrote back to the university for more details, but that the tutors never 'took the hint' to write more fully.

The interest taken in students and in the outcome of their field work was evidenced by the wish often expressed to hear more about their subsequent progress. The 'one way process' referred to by a family caseworker who said that good reports were 'poured in' to the universities, but they 'didn't get anything back' was reflected also by a probation officer at a meeting where seven of the staff discussed this survey and considered the rights and wrongs of showing reports on their field work to students. This officer said that if he was expected by the university to show his report to the student he thought *he* had a right to see the student's report on the agency. Another officer in the same service remarked sadly 'Nothing ever comes back to you'. A medical social worker said that she wanted to hear from the tutor whether the student had understood the work of the department and gained what she wanted, and to have the tutor's evaluation of her field work report after it had been discussed with the student. One sympathetic child care officer, realizing the pressure of time in departments with large numbers of students, thought that the students themselves might well be asked to write to the agency about the value of their experience. She also suggested that there might be annual group discussions with the students about their field work during the university year, a note of which could be sent to the agencies concerned.

Reference has been made to a number of difficulties in the field work of students from basic courses. Social workers also described methods which seemed to them satisfactory. How far these methods could be extended is one of the purposes of this Survey to consider, and this will be done in later chapters. The following example may set the stage for a more promising approach. This comes from one of the seven counties in which there was no course, but which was less distant than others. Here students were received in one agency from eight different courses, five basic, and three professional. The Children's Officer who saw many difficulties in offering suitable experience to students from basic courses, but *not* in communication, wrote:

> Regular contact is kept between staff of the agency and of the course by means of meetings of supervisors and course staff, supplemented by correspondence and telephone. A fully co-operative relationship has been established by means of which all relevant information can be obtained.

PART II

PROFESSIONAL COURSES

Sequence of field work in basic and professional courses

Most courses of professional training in the university require students to have completed a basic course, including field work. It seems reasonable to suppose that these students should undertake a considered sequence of practical work. Continuity of this kind may be worked out if both courses are in the same university, but this is often not the case for individual students; satisfactory sequence may then be partly a matter of luck. Some students for whom practical work is arranged between the two courses may have taken degrees in which practical work is not a requirement, or have had insufficient experience of the right kind; they may then be unprepared for their field work, and from the standpoint of the agency, they may indeed seem to be out on a limb. One description of this situation ran:

> They came and they went . . . they came from oblivion, and they went into oblivion . . . they did not seem to have a tutor.
>
> (Voluntary family case work. Students received from a variety of basic and professional courses.)

For students who have already entered upon professional training it is naturally expected that practice takes on new importance, and that responsibility will be shared more fully with those in the field than it is in basic courses. In the descriptions that follow, the contrast in the nature of the partnership is indeed striking. This is having an important effect upon attitudes towards the field work of all students.

A number of courses of new types started in recent years has given rise to much discussion between those concerned with professional education for social work, and this in itself has created a sense of partnership in fresh enterprise. When the Survey was launched the pioneer two year courses leading to the Certificate in Social Work or to recognition by the Central Training Council in Child Care had only received their second group of students. The university course in applied social studies had only been in existence for ten years and others were much more recent. Both these new types of courses adopted concurrent field work, hitherto only used in training for psychiatric social work.

Concurrent and block field work

In the Survey year the concurrent plan of training was followed in twenty professional courses; another six adopted it for one of their placements, involving altogether about two thirds of the total number of students. One university, and the then Probation Advisory and Training Council relied at this time largely upon block field work placements in widely scattered areas, and accounted for nearly a third of the total number of professional course students. The proportion of concurrent practical training in all the student placements at this date was about 43 per cent. By 1965 about half a considerably increased number of probation officer students were undertaking at least one period of concurrent field work.

Students from courses using block placements usually do field work in the service for which they hope to qualify; the staff of agency and course may then have special means of keeping in touch. Moral welfare workers for example (some of whom also undertake concurrent field work), are for full time periods with staff who have attended the same college and are familiar with its teaching; they meet together as past students and as colleagues to discuss the course as a whole. Tutor officers in the probation service are well known to training inspectors.

Concurrent and block patterns of training obviously lead to important differences in methods of communication between academic and field work staff. These differences are clearly reflected in the views expressed by professional organizations and field work staff to be considered later in this chapter.

The staff responsible for courses using mainly block placements put forward three main reasons in their favour, apart from practical considerations. These are:

1. Closer identification with the service is more satisfactorily achieved if the student is able to play a full part in all the work of the agency and to take responsibility for all the vicissitudes of his cases.

2. Some students much prefer to be wholly occupied in the service of their choice and for this reason are likely to profit more from full time field work. This was said to be particularly true of those who have spent some years in academic study and of certain students of mature years.

3. A good standard of scholarship can only be satisfactorily achieved on the academic side if students have uninterrupted periods of study.

Practical reasons for adopting this pattern were regarded as crucial at this time. Expansion in the number of students could not take place if all the courses were dependent upon local services. Block periods enabled use to be made of the best opportunities for practical training throughout the country.

Distant block placements involve obvious difficulties. In the attempt to overcome these problems interesting developments were taking place. In the university course it had been found necessary to make special appointments of university tutors to visit the agencies in which their students were placed in certain regions, to gather them at intervals for group teaching, and to hold monthly meetings for supervisors in these areas. Even so, the staff felt the need for closer integration of study and practice which they thought might be achieved if field work were arranged between two periods of academic study rather than at the end of the academic year. In the probation courses the training inspectors who act as tutors aim to visit all students and supervisors during the final period of practical training. During the Survey year it had not been possible to maintain this degree of consultation which has since been carried out. Arrangements are being made for more staff consultation through regional meetings of tutor officers as well as the conferences and courses at headquarters. A 'Tutor Officers' Bulletin' is being circulated as a means of keeping probation officers up-to-date with developments.

The need for consultation is therefore recognized in courses where there is more separation, both physically and in terms of learning. It was found however that in the methods used and the views expressed there was a different concept of partnership in the courses adopting concurrent training.

In these courses there is a remarkable degree of consistency in the way in which they initiate and sustain the partnership to which they attach so much importance. Survey interviews were held with the staff of half these courses—eight in the universities and five in colleges of further education; the methods described were so similar that we did not ask for further particulars in the correspondence inquiry.

The session was normally opened with a social gathering at which the supervisors met the academic staff. The chairmen of committees and chief administrative officers were sometimes included.

It is common practice to send supervisors some account of each main lecture course including book lists. In one university, supervisors were invited to attend lectures given to students, but few had been able to do so.

Regular meetings with the supervisors are held throughout the session, sometimes as often as once a fortnight, and never less than once a month. The Council for Training in Social Work, regarding interchange as essential, only approves courses in which provision of this kind is made. Initial discussions tended to focus upon the introductory phases of the student's work, the aims and content of training and methods of teaching casework. Some had developed study groups with wider interests, such as principles and methods of education in which other members of the academic staff took a lead. Standards by which the progress of students could be estimated were of central interest, and the ethical principles of social work and of professional education were of common concern in some courses.

Seminars were often offered to more than one group of supervisors. The groups were sometimes divided according to the length of the supervisor's experience with students, special meetings being held for those who were taking this responsibility for the first time. Other programmes provided in different groups for supervisors who received students at the first or second phase of their training. The majority of the staff also offered seminars to other social workers invited individually with a view to increasing the number of supervisors. There were also study groups led by academic staff for any caseworkers who might be interested, with a view to benefit alike to the service and to students. Sometimes such meetings were held at considerable distance from the course centres in areas where agencies not so far involved in training might eventually take students. It was sometimes preferred that seminars should be led by staff not responsible for the course in order that study should be freed from the notion of selecting supervisors.

Meetings of all the supervisors concerned with the same group of students served the purpose not only of relating fieldwork to studies in the course, but of encouraging the staff of various agencies to compare methods and distil principles. We were told that as a result of these discussions there came to be less preoccupation with *our* students and *our* service and more concern about helping students to think in terms of meeting common human needs.

Consultation about individual students

All the agency staff were given particulars in writing about each student as well as having opportunity to discuss individuals with the tutor before field work was started. Continuity between the first and second period of field work was helped by meetings of supervisors and the passing on of reports.

Supervisors sometimes served with academic staff in interviewing candidates for training. Many were invited to read the personal records of students. The view taken about the right of the supervisor to know what the tutor knew about students was supported on the ground that 'if we regard them as colleagues, we must treat them as such'. There was concern for the rights of students; some thought that they should be consulted about the passing on of information, others that this sharing of knowledge would be rightly assumed by the students, because of the nature of the partnership.

Alarm is sometimes expressed that these methods are precious and focus too much attention on the personal attitudes of students and the details of their progress. This will always be a matter of controversy and is perhaps likely to be emphasized in new endeavours for high standards of professional education. It is in the nature of this learning that students become aware of their attitudes towards people and must come to terms with them in as far as they affect their disinterested response to human need. This had been discussed as the staff considered together the way in which the individual progress of students should be assessed, and their share in appraisal.

One test of the nature of educational partnership is the importance attached to reports on practical training in the award of the professional qualification. In some of the universities it was said that the reports were regarded as the equivalent of an examination; in all the courses the standard is essential to satisfactory completion. Discussion of achievement and joint evaluation by academic and field work staff at the end of each period of practical training was said to be leading to increased reliability of standard.

The Council for Training in Social Work appoints external 'assessors' (or examiners) for each course preparing students for the Certificate in Social Work. Each college sets its own examinations. The material available to the internal examiners and the assessors includes the supervisors' report on the student's field work, which must contain sufficient evidence of the student's performance to enable the assessors to recommend to the Council that the student should pass or fail or be referred in his field work.

Importance is also attached by the Council to a written project from each student which is regarded as a further indication of his ability to relate study and practice.

The outstanding impression gained from description of these methods was the great respect felt by academic staff for those who taught their students in the field. An immense amount of thought and time is spent in developing understanding of the demands of professional education. In spite of problems in maintaining standards there was in these descriptions a note of confidence and optimism.

Views of professional associations

Members of professional associations should be in a position to exercise considered judgement of training. Many are undertaking supervision, some are in academic posts and numbers have taken an active part with their organization in discussion of standards. They have also been students. There are however wide differences in their direct concern with training. In medical and psychiatric social work, for example, the associations take considerable responsibility for setting and maintaining the standard of field work. At the other extreme, the National Association of Probation Officers, although represented on the official training body, said that they had no official part in the arrangement of field work and so could not make any useful comment.

There was considerable agreement in the replies sent by seven organizations to questions about the relationship between the staff of courses and agencies receiving students. It is evident that the development of close consultation such as had been described in the concurrent courses is greatly welcomed. Of such consultations, the Association of Family Caseworkers wrote:

> These arrangements have proved helpful to supervisors who have formed close links between university and field staff. Supervisors have been able to enjoy the stimulus of university life which encourages the positive development of thought and practice in the field. These meetings also brought together the staff of various agencies, giving individuals a fuller understanding of the work in each placement and its effect on the student.

Others referred particularly to the value of joint meetings, individual discussions in the agency and central courses on supervision.

In spite of this appreciation some of the associations are not satisfied that communication is at present truly reciprocal. The Education Committee of the Institute of Medical Social Workers, for example, wrote:

> There is much to be achieved in bridging the gap between the class room and the field. In most courses great efforts are made to link up tutors and supervisors by means of regular supervisors' meetings and occasional visits by tutors to the agency. These contacts are all understandably student focused, and although very valuable, do not entirely keep the needs of the field vividly and freshly in the minds of teaching staff. ... Schools of social work, and their tutorial staff have made considerable efforts to disseminate their ideas on aims and methods of training, both through written reports, education committees and by personal contact. At present there is no clear way of feeding back ... what are the needs of the field.

Reciprocal understanding would be improved, in the view of several of the professional organizations, if there were more discussions between the senior staff of the agencies and the tutors. It was also suggested that much would be gained if tutors could from time to time undertake periods of field work, during which, as it was expressed, 'great efforts' would be made by the agency to make this 'a positive, renewing experience'. One organization went as far as to say that they thought this should be compulsory! The Association of County Welfare Officers, regretting that their departments play only a small part in training, suggested that newly appointed tutors should spend six months with local welfare authorities in order to 'assess the full potential' that could be offered to students, and hoped that their doors should also be open to students entering other services.

Two forward-looking suggestions were made. One, warmly supported from a number of sources was that the valuable consultations already taking place between academic and field work staff should be extended on a wider front for those concerned with all aspects of training for social work; the other, that common interest in research would increasingly bring about partnership on a sound footing.

Views of field work staff

We turn now to the opinions expressed by those who were receiving students from professional courses.

The welcome given to these students and the enthusiasm expressed about training and their share in it was evident throughout the Survey. It is true that to some extent this was influenced by the desire to attract more staff to their own service, but both senior staff and those undertaking supervision found that educational responsibility put them 'on their toes', made them more aware of their own methods and principles, and was generally beneficial to liveliness and perspective. One probation officer, contemplating these influences, said 'I almost *need* a student!'

While this attitude was generally true, there was a marked difference in the degree of enthusiasm of those who took part in the close partnership which has been described in concurrent courses and those who received students for block periods from a distance. Almost all those who had experience of both patterns of training expressed approval of the concurrent plan. It is true that in our inquiry we saw less of the field work staff who received students for block periods and were so situated as to make local consultation easy. Some of the methods described, by which tutors had more frequent meetings with those responsible for their students, had not developed at the time of the Survey year. What stands out, however, is the great importance for those in the field of a sense of identification with the course, and of regular meetings with the academic staff for the study of content and method.

The feeling of isolation which was the key-note of many of the social workers receiving students at a distance from their courses was illustrated in some of the replies to inquiries sent to rural areas. Four of the eleven agencies always saw one of the tutors about the student placed with them, in five they were only sometimes visited, and in two no tutor came. One senior officer in charge of a county service, most anxious that her agency should take a full share in professional training, said that one of her staff had travelled 150 miles each way to attend an annual university meeting in the hope of achieving a closer relationship, but that this had only come about when one of her staff happened later to be appointed as a tutor to a new course, and so was completely familiar with both aspects of training. 'This isolation', she wrote, 'makes training more of a burden than it should be' and hoped that for her agency this would be remedied by the starting of a local course in a new university. Reference was made to the unsatisfactory plan of a block period of field work coming at the end of a university session, which seemed to the supervisor 'rather like an epilogue' in a training which should be 'one, rather than two, processes'.

Although efforts were made by the academic staff to convey in writing and in occasional meetings what was going on in the course, a number of those at the receiving end said they were not sufficiently aware of the changing content of courses to help the student to relate study and practice. Another comment often made was that they did not know enough about individual students and their previous training to provide them with the most suitable programme. From the courses we were told that records including reference to previous reports on practical work were always sent by tutors, but they seemed in any case to be regarded as poor substitutes for personal discussion. When tutors visited or meetings were contrived, this was evidently an occasion of great importance for supervisor, agency and student as it was in the basic courses. There was indeed consternation in some agencies about the lack of consultation with the staff of courses when students were received at a distance.

In contrast, those who worked closely with the staff of local courses spoke not only of the satisfaction, as one put it, of being 'on the same wave length' as the university, with the encouragement of 'exchanges all along the line', but the interest and illumination they gained from the meetings. To one supervisor this was 'a revelation', to another ' a very enriching business'. It seems clear that discussions acted as a fertilizer of thought, brought about insight into their own methods, and that association with colleagues in the course gave confidence. Reference was often made to the value both of personal discussion with the tutor responsible for an individual student and to consideration by all the staff of criteria of progress. Meditating about all these methods one supervisor remarked 'close contact is the nub of it all'. Nevertheless there were some reservations.

The professional associations in their evidence welcomed the close association of caseworkers with tutors, but thought there should be more consultation about the whole programme between the senior staff of agencies and courses. A few senior staff members of the agencies, including a medical officer of health, thought that these students were being given too much attention; that their supervisors were too closely identified with the educational body rather than the agency; that too much was 'taken for granted' by the training body, and that teaching might become too precious, or too 'analytical'. The amount of time given to students led to tensions in some agencies, when clinical 'teams', or students of other professions were involved.

Senior social work staff and the supervisors themselves were sometimes concerned about the amount of time spent out of the office, particularly when two sets of meetings might be attended by staff who supervised students from more than one course. The majority of the staff (based upon an estimate received from sixty-six supervisors in twenty-three agencies), were giving between sixteen and twenty hours a month; about a fifth, forty hours or more. The caseload, a notoriously misleading measure of social work, also varied greatly, a large proportion (44 per cent) fell within the range of forty-one to sixty cases, and about a fifth between sixty-one and eighty.

Most of the staff felt that the benefits of sharing in training far outweighed the strains, but that if this standard of professional education were to be maintained, time must be allowed for it by reducing work loads; there was otherwise too much conflict between their efforts to meet to the full the needs of their clients and to do justice to the students. Evidence of the value attached to meetings was that attendance was on the whole regular and that the time involved did not raise more concern. Most of the criticisms came from social workers who were too distant from the course, or too pressed for time to take advantage of meetings. One or two had written off the possibility of attendance in the second year.

Another comment made was that too much was expected in the reading and writing of reports, particularly in the early years of new courses. Reference by a supervisor to 'sheaves of stuff' which she received about the content of courses and the time-tables of students, suggested diminishing returns or individual allergy to reading duplicated papers. Some had found the writing of reports on students a heavy burden and were greatly relieved when in the second year of a new course the expected number was reduced. These and other straws in the wind suggest that eagerness for high standards sometimes defeats its own ends.

F

Field work reports are a reflection of the partnership between those who write them and those by whom they are read. There was occasional disquiet on the part of supervisors in concurrent as well as in other courses about the use made of the reports they wrote on students. Reference is made to this problem in the first Tutor Officers' Bulletin issued by the Probation Department,[1] where assurance is given that field work reports are used only in the context of training. The problem of the proper use of reports arose in a different form when agencies in which students were trained were asked to provide references for employment, sometimes before the course was completed. Some complied with this request. In one agency there had been considerable discussion about the issues raised. The decision was that the training body, to which they were committed in educational partnership, was finally responsible for records of students, and that it was not proper to separate their opinion of the student based upon a particular period of training. Differences of practice suggest that an important principle has not yet received sufficient consideration.

Views of students

Students views about the relation between their study and practice is an important test of communication between staff. Members of the Association of Social Work and Social Study students were asked the following question by their committees:

> Comment on whether you feel that there is sufficient co-ordination between your field work and theoretical training.

From students of basic courses, 64 answers were received, of which 24 (36 per cent) were satisfied with co-ordination, 32 (48 per cent) regarded it as insufficient, and the remainder did not commit themselves to either view. The following illustrations from their replies suggest great variations:

Basic Courses

F. Aged 22. Second placement. One month full time.
> Yes, definitely. Theoretical training has covered adoption, children deprived of normal home care, etc., during the term previous to the placement. My supervisor continually referred to the relevant Acts of Parliament, legislative powers of the agency and limits of the department. If all placements could be as closely linked as this one, the position would be excellent.

[1] Home Office Probation Department. Tutor Officers' Bulletin No. 1, July 1964 (unpublished).

M. Aged 23. First year. Three placements.
   No, and no again. There is no co-ordination whatsoever. No discussion of placement before or after; no mandate or tasks given; no backing for initiative.

Replies were received only from 25 students in several different types of professional courses and are not therefore representative. The following extracts from widely varied replies suggest aspects of training which seem to them to be important:

F. Aged 38. Two placements, each concurrent and partly full-time.
   Good integration between the field work and theoretical training. Supervisors have plan of lectures—discuss stage we are up to when we discuss cases. Sometimes this is self-evident by the material we present ! ! Tutor discusses one's particular cases in relation to social work theory—recommends reading relevant if they 'jump' a stage further on than theory known at that time.

F. Aged 31. Second year, third placement. Concurrent.
   Supervisors must be on the same wave-length, otherwise placement is a waste of time. Must be interested in training students. Some tutors could benefit from wider knowledge of field work (this is said with all seriousness) before presenting theory.

M. Aged 21. First year. First placement. Concurrent.
   Concurrent placements do not seem satisfactory as the student never has time to make up his mind whether he is a social worker or a student from day to day. Therefore, co-ordination seems to be lacking here.

SUMMARY AND IMPLICATIONS

The nature and degree of partnership between academic and field work staff has been considered. In basic courses there is much good will on both sides but the relationship is for the most part tenuous, not reciprocal, largely dependent upon correspondence. Many of those in the field regard this as unsatisfactory and it causes concern to a number of academic staff. If field work is to be made worth while for the coherent learning of students there is need for much more consultation between the staff of courses and agencies about its purposes and methods.

In professional courses partnership satisfactory to tutors and supervisors seems generally to be established in courses adopting concurrent field work. There is considerable dissatisfaction in the field about the placement of students for full time periods at a distance, because of comparative lack of communication; plans for closer co-operation seem likely to reduce difficulties. Communication between staff must affect training, but further study is needed to discover whether, given similar field work standards and good means of staff consultation, there are particular educational merits in concurrent and block training.

More discussion with the senior staff responsible for social services in which students are trained is essential for maintaining and extending field work of good standard.

5

STUDENT UNITS

AT the time of the Survey, staff appointments made specially for the supervision of groups of students were being extended as the number of courses and students was increased. For this and for other reasons it was important to consider their advantages and limitations. Was it for instance possible by this means to give students skilled education in the field without isolating them from the ordinary responsibilities of the service? Would this be a satisfactory way of safeguarding standards of training or might it prevent the spread of interest and competence among other social workers?

A number of practical questions are raised in the making of special appointments. What share for example is taken by the educational body on the one hand and the agency on the other in determining qualifications and financing the appointment? How extensive must the casework of the agency be in relation to the number of staff and students? How is the standard and continuity of service maintained for clients?

In this chapter we shall not consider the special arrangements sometimes made for academic staff, in co-operation with an agency, to take responsibility for teaching their own students in the field. In professional training these plans are often due to particular circumstances, such as the establishment of new types of training, or conditions at a given time in local services. Reference will later be made to a programme of field work teaching with a different purpose for students placed in a variety of agencies from basic courses (see p. 111).

Units included in this Survey

The twelve units considered in this chapter fulfilled the following conditions:

1. The appointment by a social work agency of a member of staff for the special purpose of supervising and teaching a group of students.

2. Recognition by the agency that in making this appointment the

students would have a primary claim on the time of this member of the staff whose other work was limited on this account.

3. Agreement between the staff of course and agency that students should be offered places throughout the required periods of practical training.

In most instances there was agreement between the academic staff and the agency making the appointment about the qualifications of the person to take charge of the unit.

It is not known how many such units there are. A number have been started since the Survey year and other posts are being advertised. The Advisory Council for Probation and After Care alone was responsible in 1964 for the appointment of eight senior probation officers to be in charge of units, and more have been authorized.

In three parts of the country we were told that the launching of professional courses had been almost wholly dependent upon appointments made for the supervision of student units in local services.

Sources of evidence

Discussions were held with the staff of the twelve units, nine of which were in agencies supported by public funds and three dependent upon private contribution. They included examples in a children's department, a child guidance clinic, family casework in voluntary agencies, the probation service and hospitals, including one for children and one for psychiatric patients. Half were in the provinces and half in the London area. Discussions with academic staff who sent students and with the staff of the agency where they were received enabled us in certain areas to see both sides of the picture. Opinions of academic staff in all the courses were invited by correspondence, and the same applied to professional organizations.

There was evidence from all these sources of keen interest in student units and of considerable support for them. The large majority of academic staff of professional courses were convinced that at their best units were important to the standard and extension of training; a small number were doubtful and described difficulties and limitations. The staff of basic courses were, with a few exceptions, not in favour of this kind of teaching group for their students, only a few of whom were included in the units seen. Most of the professional organizations supported the plan, but they pointed up a number of risks as well as advantages. In the agencies the units aroused mixed feelings amongst the rest of the staff.

The twelve units were studied with a view to discovering the circumstances in which they appear to flourish, the kind of risks involved, and the ways in which they affect the rest of the staff in the agencies. Their organization will first be described.

Methods of appointment

The units originated in a variety of ways. In some instances senior academic staff in the courses from which students came had taken the initiative; in others a great deal of preliminary work had been done by senior officers of the agency in consultation with those responsible for courses. National training councils had encouraged certain units and promoted discussion of their purposes and standards with the staff of the agency and the course.

Finance

Financial support of the staff appointment in nine of the twelve units came directly or indirectly from public funds. The National Health Service provides in its teaching hospitals for training responsibilities which include social work staff; the unit in the Children's Department was encouraged and subsidized by the Home Office. Two units in a voluntary family casework agency with a long tradition of student training relied, apart from small per capita fees, upon their own money raising efforts. Trust Funds met the salary of the supervisor in a second family casework organization; at the time of the Survey the period of demonstration financed from this source was coming to an end, and the future of the unit was precarious.

There was general agreement that responsibility for a training unit called for a staff member of senior status, but different views were held on whether training as such should attract an increase in salary. This is a question which relates to other supervisors and is therefore considered elsewhere. (See Chapter 6.)

Number of students and types of courses

The total number of students in these twelve units was ninety-eight, making an average of about eight students during a twelve month period. They were generally received from professional courses in two groups of three or four. In each unit some of the students were undertaking concurrent study and practice, occasionally from more than one course. The periods of field work for students on the concurrent plan were typically three days a week for four or five months, generally completed in the university courses by some weeks of full time practice. Those undertaking block periods stayed for three to four months. Two of the units included students from basic courses. The largest number of students in one unit at any given time was six.

Organization within the agency

The organization of the units is naturally related to the purpose and structure of the agency. There are obvious differences, for instance, between its place in a large hospital with a post-graduate teaching department and in a county service with area offices; between a voluntary casework agency designed partly for the purpose of training and a child guidance centre in which social work students are studying with a 'team' of psychiatrists and psychologists.

In all these varied situations it was found that the supervisor was regarded as a full member of the staff and undertook casework of her own. The units were organized in two main ways. In some instances the person in charge took over all the teaching; in others the supervision of the casework of the students was shared with other members of the staff. When the unit supervisor was entirely responsible for the casework of the students, their experience depended upon the transfer, or 'borrowing' of cases from other members of the staff; no such transfer was involved when responsibility was shared. In this case the functions of the 'senior supervisor' were to arrange the general educational programme, to decide which students were to work with different members of the staff, and to teach the students as a group. This plan meant that the supervisor acted more in the capacity of a consultant to other members of the staff. In certain psychiatric services each student is attached to a clinical team with her supervisor, and here the teaching value of the clinical unit, including psychologist and psychiatrist, is as much if not more emphasized than that of the social work unit. There were other instances of students in a unit being supervised by various members of staff; in a family casework agency each social worker had a reduced case load which allowed time to be given to one or two students.

In either case the supervisor must at all times take the final responsibility for safeguarding the interests of clients by the vigilance of her supervision and by making sure that changes from staff to student or from one student to another are properly introduced and explained.

Accommodation and clerical assistance

When a number of students work in an agency the sharing of rooms and other facilities has many repercussions. In all these twelve units separate rooms were provided both for the students and for the member of staff in charge. In nine of the offices at least one separate room was available for interviews with clients. This accommodation had not been secured without difficulty, and problems had been raised by encroachment upon space otherwise used by staff.

Clerical help is almost always available for essential case records and letters. This provision was considerably better than in the ordinary run of agencies where students are trained. The students are themselves responsible as a rule for the longer records written for educational purposes.

Methods of teaching

The fact that the programme of the unit is geared to education means that the methods used are less likely to be affected by fluctuation in pressures of work and by lack of time to make full educational use of the students' experience, both individually and in a group.

Units have sometimes been regarded as peculiar, or even as a kind of mystique, because it is thought that they employ special 'slow motion' methods of teaching casework by detailed discussion of interviewing on a few cases. These methods are of course used elsewhere, and it is important to recognize that they are not a distinguishing characteristic of units. The essential difference between teaching in a unit and other arrangements for supervision is that membership of such a group affects the range and selection of casework, encourages interchange between the students, and gives opportunity for shared teaching.

Weekly meetings for discussion with the whole group are held by the supervisor in addition to individual tutorials. The meetings appear to be used mainly for discussion of common problems of casework rather than for systematic teaching on principles and methods. The history, structure, and administration of the agency are given special attention. The senior social worker of the agency often takes over classes in which matters of policy are discussed.

General conditions for the establishment of units

There is evidence both in the history of units and in the opinions expressed about them that certain conditions are important to the fulfilment of their purposes.

It is essential that those in charge of the agency should be convinced of the value of the unit and its acceptability to the staff as a whole. There must also be a good standard of service; the unit should not be used to 'prop up' an agency suffering from staffing difficulties. In order to maintain a proper balance between the interests of clients, staff and learners a sufficiently wide range of cases is necessary. The supervisor needs to be fully identified with the agency and regarded as such. There should be reasonable assurance of the continuation of the unit for benefits to be gained.

These considerations are closely related and appear in different contexts in the descriptions that follow.

The need for continuity

It is an essential feature of units that they should regularly provide for a given number of students in relation to particular courses. Reasonable security in the arrangements is therefore one of the first considerations. In two units included in this survey the loss of staff at an early stage meant that harassed tutors had either to curtail the number of students, or to use other placements under duress. The vulnerability of units depending upon a single appointment raised one of the main doubts about their desirability. 'If the present supervisor leaves', said one tutor, 'the chances of getting a replacement are not very strong, so you are left with four unplaced students.' Other tutors who had met with less misfortune of this kind supported units because of what was otherwise a 'chronically unstable situation', and hoped that units would counteract the rapid turnover among 'casual' supervisors. It is possible that in the long run senior appointments requiring special qualification might lead to more continuity. The risks however suggest that it would always be wise to appoint one of the staff as an 'understudy', not necessarily to take a share in all the responsibilities but to be sufficiently competent and familiar with the programme to take over in an emergency.

The unit supervisor

There was general agreement that the person appointed should be a full member of the staff of the agency and should continue to be directly responsible for some clients in addition to those entrusted to students. The phrase often used was that the supervisor should be 'rooted in the agency'. This assumes good qualifications for the work itself, to which educational skill is added.

The head of the agency

Much seemed to depend upon whether training was an accepted part of the function of the agency, as it is, for example, in teaching hospitals and in certain voluntary organizations. Student units did not stand out as peculiar if professional education was an accepted purpose so that special privileges and pressures were understood.

In any case the attitude of the senior member of the staff towards the unit and the part played by staff and students in the service as a whole was found to be of the utmost importance. Integration of the training group within the service was essential and in this the head of the agency holds a key position. Not only is she responsible for interpretation to committees and administrators, but she must keep the balance between the claims of the unit and the rest of the staff. When units came under fire, the views of the critics were usually that the students and their supervisors live in a rarified atmosphere, and are insulated from real tasks and pressures.

One head of a department referred to tensions which arose in the 'triangle' of her relationships with the unit supervisor and the staff of the course which had only been resolved by 'utter frankness all round'. Another head, feeling at first at a disadvantage, curtailed other professional activities in order to bring herself up to date with the theory of social work so that she could better understand the teaching going on in the unit. Even in teaching hospitals, where a training unit was not regarded as odd, careful steering was needed to relate the work of the unit satisfactorily to the service as a whole; this it was said, did not 'just happen'. It was important to reach clear understanding about such matters as the records kept by students, and the confidential nature of certain discussions with academic staff about their educational progress.

The following illustration given in discussion with a chief medical social worker shows the way in which the situation was met in one hospital:

> The need to have a 'supervisor of trust' was emphasized, so that if anything went wrong in the hospital because of the students she was sure that it would be quickly discussed between them. In the supervisor's day-to-day work she was left perfectly free, but kept the head of the department in touch. This head thought it important that students should feel that there was a confidential quality to discussion between the academic staff and the supervisor, and that this would be respected by the head of the department.

Emphasis has been laid in other connections upon the importance of consultation between the staff of courses and the senior staff of agencies. There is an even stronger case for this consultation about student units. The fact that they *are* a group emphasizes the privilege of students. It is valuable for the service as a whole as well as for the students' education that the head of the department should take a definite share in the training programme. There should also be regular consultation between the head and the supervisor, so that the person responsible for the service as a whole is kept fully aware of the students' activities and any problems that may arise.

The risks of units

The main doubts about student units came from professional organizations and other caseworkers within the agencies. The danger of insulation from the service was the one most often raised. Closely connected with this was the fear that students trained mainly in such groups would not be well prepared for the real conditions of their future work. These anxieties were expressed in such terms as 'artificiality'; the hazards of forming in the agency 'a group within a group'; the danger of 'lack of identification' with the service. The majority of the professional associations weighed against these risks the advantages of a skilled and experienced supervisor, and the economical use of this skill; relief from pressure; easier and perhaps more profitable communication with the staff of courses, and the opportunity for the supervisor to gain cumulative experience in educational methods and in appraisal of the students' progress.

Suggestions were made by professional organizations about the ways in which risks might be offset and benefits strengthened. The Association of Children's Officers thought that supervisors should not only be 'rooted in the agency with their own caseload', but should not hold this position too long without returning to other duties.

The County Welfare Officers Society held the view that the supervisor should first have been employed as a caseworker in the agency. The Association of Family Case workers supported the plan by which other members of the staff share in the supervision of students, partly because it seemed to them important not to deprive qualified supervisors of the opportunity to train students if they so wished, but so that in any case 'the supervisory scheme should not be in a separate compartment, but integrated into the work of the agency to guard against the isolation of students'.

Staff relationships within the agency

Some of these warnings point to the importance of staff relationships within the service. Here there were evidently sources of friction; there were also useful examples of adjustment.

It must be recognized that between the pressures of service and the standards set in professional education a degree of conflict is to be expected and may be productive. In agencies where educational aims are emphasized by the presence of a special member of staff and a group of students this conflict is more evident. Students are freed from pressure of work; busy staff may feel deprived of the luxury of time for deliberation. They may also feel at a disadvantage in relation to students because they themselves are anxious for opportunities to make progress in their work by means of study, or in some instances, to gain the qualification for which the students are working.

In this general situation particular sources of difficulty may act as triggers. Put at its simplest the allocation of rooms and telephones may give rise to irritation and represent rival claims of a more sensitive nature. The transfer of cases by staff members to students is a severe test of disinterest; to be asked to take up the threads again when students leave calls for tolerance of an unusual kind. They may rightly be concerned about continuity of service for clients to whom students have perhaps been able to give more time, and less skill.

Wisely handled it seems that these difficulties can be avoided or reduced, even when the whole of the supervision rests with the person in charge of the unit. If the staff can be identified with its purposes at the outset, if due respect is paid to their own responsibility for clients to whom the service of students is offered, and if their position as staff members is given full recognition, the unit should result in gains for the agency as a whole.

In a Children's Department, for example, where a number of difficulties had been experienced, certain changes were made. Here the appointed supervisor was entirely responsible for teaching students in the unit. Importance was attached to opportunities for study for other members of the staff, which became the responsibility of the deputy. Some of the seminars offered by the university were open to any staff members. A clear distinction was made between the purposes of meetings in which staff and students discussed together and those in which students were not included. When cases were transferred the student was personally introduced to clients by the child care officer.

Taking risks and benefits into consideration there seems much to be said for the pattern of unit in which other members of the staff also supervise the casework of one or two students and look to the person in charge for consultation. The possibilities of a plan of this kind depend however on a number of conditions, including the structure and function of the agency and the qualifications and experience of other members of the staff. In county services, where casework staffing and transport are suitable, the advantages of supervision in different area offices might well be combined with the teaching of the group at headquarters.

Views of staff and students working in units

Support for units, as one might expect, came from all those in charge of them, and this was true even of one member of staff who herself expressed preference for individual teaching. Professional associations confirmed some of the advantages: easy and helpful communication with the staff of courses, and gains made by steady practice of teaching. One supervisor put it 'a unit is a means of teaching supervisors to teach'. This applied both to their work with individuals and with the group. Cumulative experience with a number of students made them less exercised about the progress of certain individuals, and more confident in their assessments. We were told by several experienced academic staff that their reports on students showed more balanced judgement. Clear recognition of their responsibility for training was said to relieve them of feeling torn between the claims of students and clients. Group teaching was regarded as valuable in itself, and also economical in the use of time given to the discussion of certain topics. The students gained from discussion of their varied experiences and also from letting off steam with one another. One of the supervisors described such a unit as being 'richer in learning and support' than other arrangements for field work.

It might be thought that there would be too much overlap between the supervisor and the academic staff in what was taught, particularly about the principles and practice of case work, but there was no hint of this in the discussions held with both.

The test of units as a method of professional education lies of course in the quality of service of those who train in them. This was beyond the scope of the Survey, but the comments of students and of some recently qualified medical social workers give some reflection of the views of those who trained in groups.

The students' comments referred only to whether or not they preferred to work in an agency with other students or on their own and not to units as such. The majority of the fifty-eight who had both kinds of experience were from basic courses, and this situation is of course different from the units described. It is however worth noting that there were very few students who did not prefer working with others rather than being placed by themselves. They referred particularly to the fact that it was helpful to pool experiences and to share mutual problems in the discussions they had with the supervisor and among themselves. On the other hand there were some opinions rather emphatically expressed about the merits of being an only student, 'able to mix with the staff and never referred to as a student'; 'personal contact with the staff easier'; (in a group) 'felt more "studenty" and less able to take up responsible attitude'. This perhaps bears out the view expressed by the Association of Family Caseworkers that 'certain students seem to benefit from a particular one-to-one relationship with a supervisor . . . and some tend to be inhibited in a group'.

In the evidence of forty-three recently trained medical social workers[1] two views were given by the majority. One was the increased value of learning together, both with their supervisor and in their own group; the other, that while they were aware of the danger of insulation most of them thought that this could be prevented. The views of a minority illustrated the risks already considered.

Two correspondents supporting units expressed their views in the following way. Both had trained in a hospital unit:

> This plan has an essential value in that it enables an agency to take several students, which with the overall shortage of student placements, is an important consideration. I feel that the benefit obtained by any individual student in this sort of placement is naturally related very directly to the student's needs, both personal and professional. I do not feel a group becomes an artificial one and a certain amount of group support can be of value. In order not to limit the benefits of the student's contacts with other members of the staff, it is, I think, essential that the whole agency is involved in, and interested in, the student group and that the supervisor herself is an integral part of the agency.

> I believe the appointment of a special member of staff with specific duties of teaching and supervision, and with only a small caseload, has a great deal to recommend it, although presumably this is only possible in a large department or agency . . . I think felt we that it was an advantage to have a supervisor who not only had sufficient time to spare from her other duties, but who was, in addition, an excellent and willing teacher. I found that students in other placements tended to be used rather more as additional staff in an overworked agency; also it does not necessarily follow that a good and well qualified social worker will make a good teacher. Incidentally, teaching in small groups helps to overcome the limitations of a

---

[1] It so happened that these individual notes from medical social workers came directly to the Survey staff, while other comments from their recently trained members were summarized by professional organizations (see p. 140).

very small caseload, as students will inevitably discuss their cases among themselves and so learn from each other. I do not think that the teaching in small groups need be unduly artificial and I believe it is up to the supervisor to encourage and facilitate contact between other members of the staff and the students.

The importance of the part played by the head of the department and by staff meetings is illustrated in the following answer which also came from experience of a hospital unit:

In the unit, in addition to individual supervision, we had a regular period each week for discussion in a group on any matter affecting our work (it was up to us to decide what we wanted to talk about), meetings with the head almoner and, towards the end of our time, opportunity to attend the departmental staff meeting. There were plenty of opportunities for meeting other members of the staff over tea and lunch. It was a great relief to have other students to give one moral support and to have an identity in the department as 'the students'. I think, too, that certainly as far as an institution like a hospital is concerned, it is easier for other personnel to cope with a unit than an individual. The unit can be fitted into the scheme of things, and its function be recognized, apart from the individual personalities making it up, whilst where there is only one, the lines often blurred and the training function gets confused with other issues.

Some of the risks involved and the different ways in which they may be presented are illustrated in the following comment made by a medical social worker who had recent experience as a student, both in a family casework agency and in a hospital:

I think there are obvious advantages for the training body and supervisors concerned, if special supervisors are appointed. Coordination is facilitated, and the training body can more easily ensure uniformity of standards and principles among the workers responsible for students. With so much pressure upon the supervisors, they can consolidate over a period their collected experience of the teaching process, with benefit to themselves and students alike.

I think there is danger that such a group of students and special supervisors becomes precious and artificial, and limits the student's experience of the wider implications of the setting. The extent to which this happens is partly controllable by the staff of the unit concerned—very often students work on cases 'borrowed' from other members of the department and this may be a useful point of contact. One disadvantage of insufficient contact between students and members of a department, is that the student has even less opportunity than usual to study the working of a department. In one agency I worked in as a student, we gained a great deal of knowledge about the unit, and met other members of the staff by attending the regular staff meetings at which new cases referred to the agency were discussed. I recognized that in many departments this would not be feasible, particularly at meetings in which matters of department policy are under discussion.

Student units in Scotland

It was interesting to find some confirmation of these findings in Scotland, where units were discussed with the staff of courses and also with supervisors in a variety of services. At this time there were only two units, corresponding to the definition in this chapter, both of which were in hospitals. A third in a family casework agency was staffed by a tutor of a professional course. The summary of these interviews ran:

> The general impression gained was that the courses favour units as a means of affording them quality placements on which they would have first call. The close working which results between tutors and supervisors helps the integration of theory and practice and mutual understanding of each other's standards of assessment is fostered. On the other hand, a number of supervisors not working in units felt that there was a danger that this method of providing field experience tended to protect the student from some of the pressures to which they will inevitably be subjected when responsible for their own workload as a member of a busy department.

One important question raised was whether the spread of student units might discourage the appointment of training officers for the purpose of staff development and in-service training.[1] These responsibilities are not incompatible; in the right setting they should prove complementary. In-service opportunities for study are essential to progress in any social service. The training of students should always be seen both by students and staff as preparation for continued learning in employment.

It is sometimes said that concentration of students will prevent the spread of interest and competence in field work training. It is not

[1] See Moscrop, Martha E. *In Service Training for Social Agency Practice.* Toronto University Press, 1958.

suggested in this chapter that units can or should provide an answer for most courses, agencies or students. None the less in proper conditions the support they are receiving seems to justify units as one useful means of progress in educational methods and in the extension of satisfactory field work for an increasing number of students.

The staff who said that the unit must be 'rooted in the agency' recognized an important truth. The site and the gardeners need to be chosen with care if the plants of education and of service are both to flourish. Good gardening depends upon knowledge, foresight, and unremitting care.

SUMMARY AND IMPLICATIONS

This study of twelve student units involving special appointments to agencies, gives empirical evidence of their value, provided there is reasonable guarantee of continuity, and that careful attention is paid to conditions in which they are established and developed. Considerations of importance are the standard, and scale of the agency; conviction of its value by senior staff; full commitment of the supervisor to the responsibilities of the service to clients; respect for the interests and professional progress of other members of the staff. There is otherwise risk of insulation.

In some agencies there are likely to be benefits if responsibility for supervision is shared with other members of the staff. There is in any case need for experiment and comparative study.

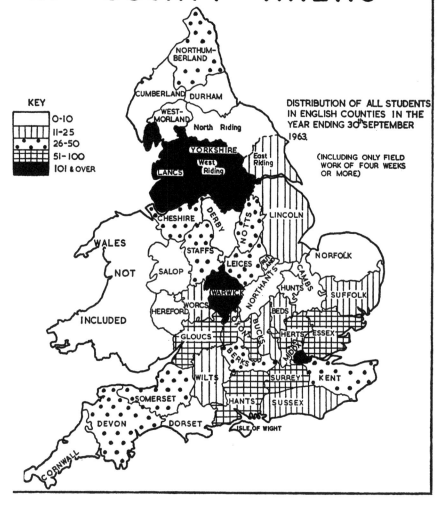

ENGLAND
STUDENT PLACEMENTS
IN COUNTY AREAS

KEY

	0-10
	11-25
	26-50
	51-100
	101 & OVER

DISTRIBUTION OF ALL STUDENTS IN ENGLISH COUNTIES IN THE YEAR ENDING 30ᵗʰ SEPTEMBER 1963.

(INCLUDING ONLY FIELD WORK OF FOUR WEEKS OR MORE)

NORTHUMBERLAND
CUMBERLAND
DURHAM
WEST-MORLAND
North Riding
YORKSHIRE
East Riding
West Riding
LANCS
CHESHIRE
DERBY
NOTTS
LINCOLN
WALES NOT INCLUDED
STAFFS
SALOP
LEICES
RUTLAND
NORFOLK
WARWICK
NORTHANTS
HUNTS
CAMBS
SUFFOLK
WORCS
HEREFORD
BEDS
GLOUCS
OXON
BUCKS
HERTS
ESSEX
MDDX
BERKS
WILTS
SURREY
KENT
SOMERSET
HANTS
SUSSEX
DEVON
DORSET
ISLE OF WIGHT
CORNWALL

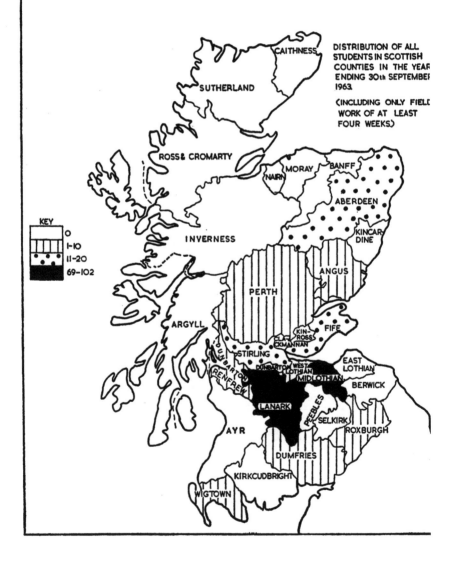

SCOTLAND
STUDENT PLACEMENTS
IN COUNTY AREAS

DISTRIBUTION OF ALL
STUDENTS IN SCOTTISH
COUNTIES IN THE YEAR
ENDING 30th SEPTEMBER
1963.

(INCLUDING ONLY FIELD
WORK OF AT LEAST
FOUR WEEKS)

KEY

O — 0
|||| — 1-10
•••• — 11-20
■ — 69-102

CAITHNESS
SUTHERLAND
ROSS & CROMARTY
MORAY
NAIRN
BANFF
ABERDEEN
KINCAR-DINE
INVERNESS
ANGUS
PERTH
KIN-ROSS
CLA-CKMANNAN
FIFE
ARGYLL
STIRLING
DUNBARTON
WEST LOTHIAN
EAST LOTHIAN
RENFREW
MIDLOTHIAN
BERWICK
LANARK
PEEBLES
SELKIRK
AYR
ROXBURGH
DUMFRIES
KIRKCUDBRIGHT
WIGTOWN

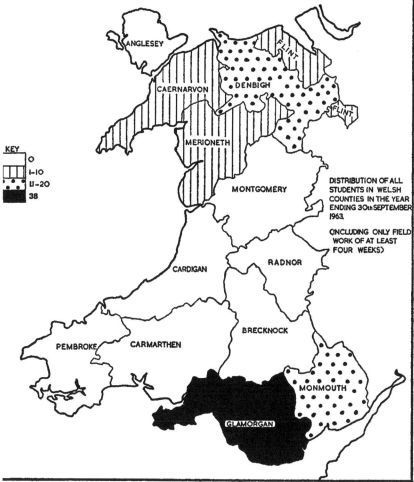

6

EXPANSION OF FIELD WORK

THERE are four main ways in which opportunities for field work might be extended. These are:

1. Further geographical distribution in areas not fully used
2. Widening the range of agencies and centres in which students are placed
3. Co-ordination between training bodies for the consideration of field work priorities for students from different types of courses
4. Grouping students so that some teaching in the field can be shared.

All these methods of extension depend upon engaging to the full the interest and support of those in charge of services; upon giving educational help to the staff, and providing the best possible means for easing unessential pressures.

1. *Geographical distribution*

Maps of the placement of students throughout the country in a twelve month period show very uneven distribution. Although in the Survey year there was consultation in regions between those promoting courses and the staff of certain services, there was no way in which the concentration of students in any one city or county could be known except by specific inquiry to each inspectorate or agency. Indeed in relation to some courses and services it was as though instead of using time tables, prospective passengers were each to go to the station to find out what trains passed that way and the vacancies they were likely to have for travellers.

It was not surprising, therefore, to find that although students were being refused for certain courses partly or wholly because of lack of suitable field work, there were counties to which for no obvious reason very few students went. The figures relate to students who were sent for periods of at least four weeks. Out of forty-eight English county areas there were thirteen in which fewer than ten students had been received. In county boroughs with a population of at least 100,000, this was true of thirty-two out of forty-seven. There were thirteen in which there had been only one student or none at all. The maps of Scotland and Wales suggest even greater contrasts.

Geographical distribution is of course affected by the adoption of the concurrent plan of field work in most of the new courses. Local opportunities in relation to new courses are explored by councils promoting professional training but there is no evidence that those who are making plans for students from *basic* courses have comprehensive knowledge of social services suitable for students all over the country; indeed, the setting up of new courses, while adding considerably to information about certain local resources, has made it still more urgent to explore further afield.

There are likely to be good reasons why students are not placed in certain areas, some of which are obviously geographical. Scattered population and poor transport in some parts of the country may present insuperable difficulty, or may be made impossible through limits placed on the use of cars. This does not seem, however, to account for differences found between other counties.

2. *The use of a wider range of agencies and centres*

The concentration of students from professional and basic courses on certain casework agencies had already been described (See Tables IIA and B, and Chapter 2). The use of *new* types of casework service for the training of professional students, in view of the criteria of choice, is only likely to take place gradually, particularly if they are dependent upon local agencies, though more opportunities for all these students are likely to develop with the increasing co-ordination of local authority services for families. It is surprising that such a small proportion of students from professional courses were gaining experience in community care, in view of the extension of this service in medical and psychiatric social work.

If the range of experience could be extended for students from basic courses the position might be eased in a number of ways. It has been seen that the academic staff want their students to have experience which broadens their knowledge of ordinary living conditions. It is therefore surprising to find, for example, that only two students were placed in services for the elderly; that only four were spending any substantial time in housing departments; and that, apart from the London school care committees, a trivial number were attached to school services for children. Again, apart from residential work few ways seem to have been found of giving these students experience with handicapped persons. Does this suggest scope for enterprise in these fields, if necessary with additional supervision provided?

In order to get some indication of trends in the choice of field work the staff of all courses were asked whether any new *types* of experience had been arranged for their students in the year following that of the survey (1963-4). Over two-thirds of the twenty-five basic courses had planned what were for them new departures, but with a few exceptions these students went along well trodden paths. This was also in the main true of replies on the *increased* use of agencies in which students had already been placed. Two features of interest emerged. One was the increase in the number and variety of placements in or related to residential care and treatment, which in both replies headed the list. The other was that a few more students were being placed in New Towns or were taking part in rural surveys. It was also of interest that British as well as overseas students were gaining various kinds of experience in other countries.

These trends were illustrated in comments made by academic staff about the ways in which they would like to extend opportunities for their students. For example:

> I should like to see more emphasis in basic courses in encouraging students to consider their individual clients against the background of their jobs, leisure groups, the communities in which they live, etc., and think they should be encouraged to develop a more anthropological interest in and acceptance of all sorts and kinds of people and ways of life . . . (but) we have difficulty in finding satisfactory community development and group work vacancies.
>
> (University: degree, one year post-graduate and
> two year non-graduate courses.)

Residential experience

Residential experience was arranged for most of the students in rather more than a third of the courses, and occasionally in all the rest. (See Table III.) Children's homes and approved schools accounted for 63 per cent of these placements; recuperative centres and prisons were being increasingly used. Few students are placed in the large number of homes for adults, such as those for the elderly or handicapped. Comment about this was received from the County Welfare Officers' Society who wrote that as far as they knew only three counties had been approached about placing social work students in their 'abundant' establishments. Heavy demands upon homes and approved schools

TABLE III
PLACEMENTS IN RESIDENTIAL WORK
BASIC AND PROFESSIONAL COURSES

Number of student placements for four weeks or over ('long') and under four weeks ('short') in England, Scotland and Wales during the year 1 October 1962 to 30 September 1963

TYPE OF INSTITUTION	COURSES							
	BASIC AND PROFES-SIONAL		BASIC			PROFESSIONAL		
	No.	%	Number long	short	%	Number long	short	%
TOTALS	588	100	179	117	100	116	170	100
Approved Schools	115	19·6	36	29	22·0	8	42	17·5
Borstal Institutions	26	4·4	4	7	3·7	2	13	5·2
Children's Homes	257	43·7	80	66	49·3	59	52	38·9
Handicapped Persons (adults and children)	46	7·8	17	4	7·1	8	17	8·7
Hospitals (nursing assis. or orderly)	4	0·7	2	2	1·3			
Hostels and Homes (adults)	6	1·0	1		0·3	2	3	1·8
Maternity or Mother and Baby Homes	23	3·9	2		0·7	12	9	7·3
Old People's Homes	21	3·6	5	2	2·4	8	6	4·9
Prisons	17	2·9	6	5	3·7	1	5	2·1
Probation Homes and Hostels	8	1·3	4		1·3	3	1	1·4
Psychiatric Care	7	1·2	3		1·0	3	1	1·4
Recuperative, Moral Welfare, Rehabilitation	51	8·7	18	2	6·8	10	21	10·8
Work Camps	1	0·2	1		0·4			
Unclassified	6	1·0						

for children are already made for students qualifying for residential work.

There was evidence from academic staff and students that under satisfactory conditions and with adequate preparation residential experience has particular value. It calls for immediate personal response different in nature from casework; provides a means of getting to know people by doing things *with* them, and, in the face of continual demands, of learning to stand the test of daily living. Students who may not at present study group relations at least experience their impact. Some institutions provide a useful example on a small scale of administrative plans and problems. For certain services residential work is a requirement for qualification so that social workers and residential staff will better understand one another's responsibilities when they later become colleagues.

Although the large majority of the students valued this experience there were a number of instances in which the lack of a programme of work or of opportunities for discussion made it much less revealing than it would otherwise have been.

The values and some of the difficulties were illustrated by staff and students. Both the following views come from the staff of large university departments offering all types of basic courses:

> Residential work gives a unique opportunity for getting alongside people and learning to understand and appreciate them, and also a chance to learn about stresses and strains of residential work and to appreciate the contribution of staff. It can also give an opportunity to learn about administration and to study relationships within a group.
>
> I have found the experience gained almost always valuable, though occasionally in a negative rather than a positive sense . . . very varied even in the same type of Home or Institution, as so much depends on personal characteristics and attitudes of staff. (After referring to special values of classifying schools and reception centres). Prisons offer a wide variety of experience, also for more mature students, e.g. to work with the Welfare Officer, or to work in workshops alongside the prisoners, or to work with the prison staff as a temporary 'extra'.

Students

The following illustrations were given by young students undertaking two to three weeks residential work during a one year postgraduate basic course.

Hostel for maladjusted children

I found my stay in the hostel valuable because I was helped to enter fully into the life of the community and felt I was of use. I learnt much from this practical experience of life in the hostel. I was also given every opportunity to discuss questions with members of the staff, and outside visits were also arranged for me . . . I felt I was not 'over supervised' and was given a considerable measure of freedom and responsibility. However, I did feel I could appeal for help at any time and all my questions were answered as fully as possible.

Prison

The value of this period was in the fact that I had complete freedom to go everywhere in the prison and talk to everyone. Hence I got to know a lot about the working of the prison and the feelings of both staff and inmates. However I feel it would be better if a student was attached to one person on the staff and was able to do something by way of work however menial.

But in contrast, cryptically, after experiences in an establishment for young people:

Unpleasant, but very salutary. Excellent stimulus for critical faculties. Supervision: 'nil'.

Exploring new resources

It was to explore possibilities of expansion, both in geographical distribution and types of experience that a county was chosen for special study. Area III, as it will be called, was taken as an example of the thirteen counties in which fewer than ten students had been placed.

Nine students had been received in this county during the Survey year. The population was between 800,000 and 900,000, including one county borough of about 105,000. The chances of training developments taking place were better here than in some other counties with similar population, social services and public transport. Three universities and two colleges of further education lay within sixty miles of the county borough and between them provided eleven courses for social workers, five basic, six professional. Although recently an occasional student from two professional courses had travelled between thirty and fifty miles for weekly field work, it was recognized that this journey in addition to social work visits in the county, involved considerable strain. The supervisors had managed to reach fortnightly meetings at course centres. Other social workers had during the past year taken part with enthusiasm in a series of seminars offered by a member of the staff of a university professional course, without commitment on either side to future supervision of students. There was evidence of increasing co-operation between the staff of public and voluntary social services; a useful county list of public and voluntary services had been printed. The county residential college of further education had welcomed overseas students of social work and education for whom a yearly programme introducing them to the life and social services of the area had been designed.

Rapid expansion of population employed in the major industry had led to an early New Town Development Corporation and to the need for social services to meet the characteristic problems of an 'immigrant' labour population. These problems had given rise to consultation between the staff concerned with personal welfare in this industry, with housing, community development and certain casework services.

In exploring the resources of this county we had in mind three questions:

1. What was the attitude of the staff towards undertaking the supervision of students?

2. Had opportunities been used as they arose or was there evidence of lack of communication with the staff of courses?

3. Were there suitable openings for experience or training of a kind seldom used, and if so how might these be developed?

There was no doubt about the interest in the training of students of almost all the senior staff. In the social services where they were occasionally received the staff wanted to have them more regularly and to consider future plans of training, as they expanded their establishment and improved their accommodation. In social organizations in which no students had been received, keen interest was expressed, including the 'personal relations' department of a major industry, an urban district council housing department, local authority health, welfare and education departments, and hospitals.

Why were these opportunities not more fully used? Certain of the agencies had been under review by training bodies promoting courses for particular services, and they may have had good reasons for deciding not to place students at any given time. In other cases opportunities no longer used for professional courses might have been of value for students from basic courses had it been known that they were available. There were, for example, three casework agencies where the changed pattern of professional training meant that students were no longer sent; arrangements had been brought to an end in one case when field work became concurrent and in another when students were placed mainly in units. The staff of these agencies had been puzzled and discouraged by changes of policy. Since the Survey year occasional approaches from courses were being made, partly because of the influence of the seminars.

It was not possible in this brief study to judge to what extent satisfactory supervision might be extended, but it seemed that all the casework agencies with experience of supervision could with good planning take more students, and that a few useful openings could be offered in departments and casework agencies not hitherto used. Additional staff appointments in three large agencies may soon bring considerable changes, and this points to the need for continuing information.

The study of this county suggested four main ways in which opportunities for field work might be expanded in similar, relatively unused areas:

(a) Periodic review from the training standpoint of all social services.

(b) The possibility of establishing a unit for students of professional courses for whom block periods of training are required.

(c) Review of agencies not well suited for professional training in which students from basic courses might be supervised, possibly supported by a staff appointment for supplementary teaching.

(d) An experiment of a field study centre in a New Town. Here students placed in a variety of settings such as the personnel department of the major industry; the housing departments, youth employment services, schools and modern community centres might bring together their studies for educational discussion.

3. *Co-ordination between training councils and between courses*

Such plans would clearly mean the pooling of certain kinds of information and more central and regional consultation between those who promote and those who organize courses. Three-quarters of the academic staff and all except one of the professional associations urged the need for such consultation in the use of scarce resources. Running through the comments made by the academic staff there is, however, anxiety that bureaucracy might creep in to formalize, limit, complicate or deaden the partnership between the staff of courses and agencies. Further apprehension was expressed, when, partly for the sake of testing its strength, academic staff were asked to say whether they thought there was a case for special 'consultants', independent of courses or agencies, to help in the development of supervised field work. This proposal raised definite opposition, though it had some supporters, and it is understood that one of the national training councils had thought the plan worth consideration.

Co-ordination between courses in the arrangement of field work received more general and emphatic support from the professional associations, and examples were given of its value in certain regions. The Association of Psychiatric Social Workers, in some ways less likely to suffer from shortage of supervision because of the history of training for this service, wrote:

> The need for some central or regional planning of the use of scarce field work placements is essential. . . . Some courses retain placements without any discussion of the urgent needs of other courses in the area and this is considered most unsatisfactory.

This Association referred to an area in which representatives of all the organizations concerned with training proposed to meet to discuss the placement of both groups of students with the Institute of Medical Social Workers.

The Association of Child Care Officers urged the importance of involving the *agencies* in consultations which took place between the staff of courses:

> Certain agencies because of their function, focus, staff structure and methods, can cater for the particular needs of certain students at different stages of training. We feel that this should be accepted clearly and made generally known so that the agencies are able to accept their own situation and put it to common use. It is felt that there should be clear thinking, and honest talking. It should be recognized that from time to time, because of staff and policy changes, what a department can offer to the training of students will change.

The Institute of Medical Social Workers added emphatic support, and raised the main practical problem:

> There have been 'gentleman's agreements' between training bodies, and some effort by schools to obtain direct information from more or less 'local' agencies, but there is a great need for some co-ordination to ensure the best use of all available place-ments. The situation is an ever changing one, and needs to be kept constantly under review. This is a sizeable job, and the question is, who is to undertake it?

This is indeed a pertinent question. Care would have to be taken to keep facts up to date, easy to assemble and to use.

4. Grouping students for field work teaching

The case for student units and the influences and conditions which seem necessary to gain advantages and avoid mistakes have been considered in Chapter 5. There are, of course, other ways in which some group teaching for students in the field can be provided by academic staff or by special educational appointments serving staff and students in a variety of agencies. Area III provided an example of a setting in which there seemed promise for experiments of this kind.

There would seem to be advantages in the development in certain casework agencies of special programmes of experience and study of a different kind for students from basic and from professional courses; such a plan is implied in the comment of the Association of Child Care Officers. It was however put to us by some academic and senior social work staff that it is important in the expansion of training to use the varied educational abilities of social workers in the same agency with students at different stages in their courses. Some senior staff in the field regarded the experience with beginning students as a means of developing the skill needed for those at the professional stage. Others thought that these educational tasks were equally skilled, though different in kind. Certainly if methods of field work teaching were to fulfil some of the aims described by academic staff, very skilled teaching would be needed in the field for students from basic as well as from professional courses. In any case, the fact that most of the staff at both ends see the need for different methods suggests that special programmes in the field need to be devised.

One such experiment, supervised by a university teacher, has provided educational experience in succeeding years for degree students through a continuing study of a rural community. Settlements, as their purposes in the community are redefined, are offering valuable programmes of neighbourhood study, used for a substantial number of students from basic courses. Another experiment[1] for supplementing the teaching of students placed in a variety of casework agencies seen during the course of the Survey provided an example of the possibility of expansion if, in certain areas, special appointments were made.

This scheme provides for a full-time appointment of a professionally qualified social worker known as a 'Teaching Caseworker'. His job is to act as co-ordinator of a programme for students placed in a variety of agencies from a number of basic courses. Regular classes are held with the students and their supervisors are offered consultation if they wish. During a ten year period financed from Trust Funds the scheme

[1] University of Sheffield and Sheffield Council of Social Service.

was extended from two agencies to most of the main voluntary and public casework services of the city; the number of places for students expanded from four to thirty, and the number of supervisors increased from thirteen to twenty-three. In 1964, students were coming from eight courses in all parts of the country. Stress is laid upon the importance of direct relationship between the staff of the agency and the staff of each course in arrangements made for individual students and reports on their work. The Teaching Caseworker is, however, increasingly consulted by the staff of agencies and courses so that opportunities are well used. Seminars are arranged not only for those who are supervising the students but for other caseworkers in the area. The supervisors share in weekly classes both on principles of social work, and to discuss the students' own presentation of cases from a variety of agencies.

Within this group, in contrast to many of the situations discussed in agencies where students are scattered, agreement seemed to have emerged on certain aims in an eight-week period, said to correspond closely with those being prepared by the Joint University Council:

1. To illustrate the teaching of social administration (i.e. to achieve in the student a better understanding of social needs and conditions, and of services available to meet them, than is possible by a purely academic study);

2. to give the student an opportunity to test himself in a casework situation;

3. to promote objective thinking, even when feelings are aroused;

4. to assess the student's reliability and responsibility, ability to adapt to new situations, and to form constructive working relationships;

5. to understand clients' reactions to services and to a wide range of personal needs;

6. to observe and participate in a variety of services and to compare the different forms of administration, structure and procedures relevant to different purposes; and to realize something of the professional competence, attitudes and practices appropriate to the services.[1]

The success of this scheme for university students seems to depend upon the confidence of the agencies in the teacher as a practitioner, and his recognition by the university for academic courses. The field work tutor himself supervised students in a family casework agency, but the

---

[1] Quoted by kind permission from the memoranda of the Sheffield scheme.

experiment seemed to show that it was important for the person in charge not to be closely identified with any particular agency. In 1964 the local authority made a financial contribution to the scheme for a three year period in order that the health and welfare services (not previously offering casework experience) could be included.

Means of encouraging expansion

Directions for general expansion have now been considered. Opinions were expressed about certain essential measures which will now be discussed before drawing conclusions.

Enlisting the support of senior administrative staff

Senior officers are responsible for interpretation to committees, and extended training depends upon their interest and sanction. Recent emphasis upon the teaching of casework has led to much more consultation between academic staff and the supervisors of their students than with heads and deputies responsible for the social services. This fact reflects confidence in the training partnership authorized, and for the most part readily supported by senior staff.

Some comments, however, suggested uneasiness—for example, 'my staff seem now to belong to the university'. The interest of senior staff in an educational programme including problems of policy and administration was often not enlisted. An illustration was given by a senior officer with sixteen years' experience of training students in a local authority department and in full accord with the advance of casework methods, in which a considerable programme of teaching on administration had been dropped. It had become accepted that he was only 'a provider' for students, not involved in their training.

Extension of field work in terms of the number of students and the wider use of agencies seems to involve a different approach to those who are responsible for the services. Some of the academic staff have become increasingly aware of this. It was also emphasized in the views expressed by the professional associations, six out of seven seeing this as a problem needing special attention. Their statements show vividly how it appears from the standpoint of the agency:

> Committees and Boards of Governors should accept some responsibility for social work training, but they cannot do this unless they are kept informed and up-to-date in plans for students' training. There is need for two-way communication here which is often ignored.
> (Institute of Medical Social Workers' Education Committee.)

We believe that the present non-involvement of Committees and Departments is not due to any reluctance on their part but rather to lack of opportunities for them to play an effective role in training their future staff.

(County Welfare Officers Society.)

Too often the casework and administrative functions of an agency are two separate warring sections rather than being indivisible and dependent on each other. Exclusion leads to suspicion and often the administrator can be made to feel that something is going on in his department about which he knows very little. By being asked actively to participate in students' training he would in time gain some understanding of the caseworker and of the rather peculiar needs of casework teaching. It is clear that more thought must be given to the mechanics of how administrative officers can be involved in training.

(Association of Family Case Workers.)

A more satisfied point of view in this regard, illustrative of centrally organized training for a specific service, came from the National Association of Probation Officers:

Principal Probation Officers and the Home Office Inspectorate endeavour to gain the interest and support of Probation Committees for the training of students . . . (they) would normally meet the principal officer in any area and have opportunities to understand administrative problems.

The Association of Directors of Welfare Services gave a useful indication of the way in which concern for training might be further developed from the standpoint of senior administrators. They considered it essential that:

Chief Administrative Officers and members of committees display an active and sustained interest in all matters connected with the training of students. The willingness of members of the Association to display this interest is apparent but there is evidence that this interest has not always been fostered by those responsible for courses. There are some complaints of ignorance amongst tutors of Local Authority Administration. The 'Chief Officer Weeks' of the National Institute for Social Work Training are welcomed for the stimulation they offer to the formation of informed attitudes towards training.

Extended study for caseworkers

Throughout this Survey it has been said in no uncertain terms and in spite of many problems that the services as well as the students stand to gain by the educational responsibilities of the staff. This suggests that there would be wide support for the further development of programmes of study for supervisors and of in-service training for staff.

In Area III much interest had been aroused and some openings for students developed in this and in another relatively 'unused' area to which the tutor of a professional course travelled throughout the university session. There were also encouraging examples of co-operation between the staff of courses in universities and colleges of further education in sharing responsibility for seminars attended by field workers who were or who might later be concerned with students from either course.

National training councils and some professional bodies offer short full-time courses on supervision, mainly, but not always for the staff of their own services. The Home Office Advisory Council for Probation and After-care provides tutor-officer courses; residential sandwich courses have for many years been arranged by the Central Training Council in Child Care and are being increased. Distinguished teachers from the United States and from Canada have played an important part in seminars designed for staff of various services. The sharing of such courses seems on all counts to be a fruitful means of progress.

The extension of these opportunities was warmly supported but there were warning notes from some academic staff of professional courses about the form they should take. There was some apprehension about the study of supervision as 'a thing in itself'; discussion of educational method should, it was thought, be based upon first hand experience with students and there were added advantages if these discussions related to supervision being undertaken at the time, as it is in concurrent courses. According to this view those who might later supervise students must first learn to appraise their own methods.

One of the academic staff reflected this view when she wrote:

> I doubt whether their first need is to study methods of training—the eternal problem of supervisors is to keep up to date with new knowledge belonging to the *content* of courses (including field work content), and the content of practice. If supervisors know what they should teach, they can study the 'how' more effectively.

Finance: students, supervisors and agencies

In Chapter 3 it was shown that the choice of field work for students from basic courses is sometimes arbitrarily affected by disparities of grant. Publicity has been given to the difficulties experienced by students of professional courses because of additional costs involved in their field work. Mature students with family responsibilities, of whom there are likely to be increasing numbers, raise special financial problems. In some areas inadequate mileage allowances for cars have prevented suitable placements from being used. There was evidence of a generous attitude on the part of agencies towards meeting difficulties of transport when these arose, but some were worried by the different arrangements for individual students, and occasionally embarassed by the hardship of those who had to wait unduly for reimbursement of expenses from public funds. These considerations are important if field work is to be satisfactorily extended into all areas of the country.

The cost of practical training to public bodies and particularly to voluntary agencies is giving rise to much discussion and bears upon what has already been said about the full engagement in the training programme of those who are responsible for the service. Senior staff must cost and support expenditure on students in terms of salary, time and accommodation. This has been a critical question when agencies are asked to make additional appointments for student units, or to reduce the work load of staff to give them time for supervision.

Two main issues are involved. One is whether training responsibilities should, as such, call for a special rate of salary or increment; the other where the cost of student training in the field properly lies.

Medical and psychiatric social workers responsible for students are entitled to a negotiated scale. It is usual for staff in other agencies to be appointed at a higher rate on the salary scale if they are taking considerable responsibility for students, particularly for training units. Voluntary organizations have based their estimate of the cost of weekly time given to students upon the assumption that members of the staff will receive a senior grade of salary.

There was considerable support from academic staff and from professional organizations for linking salary scale or special increment with responsibility for students. Five out of seven of the professional organizations held this opinion. The arguments put forward are: the importance of offering a financial incentive to caseworkers to undertake supervision; the likelihood that this recognition will lead to greater continuity of relationship with academic staff; the influence that this may have upon the quality of teaching and the time given to students. There was more divided opinion on the part of the staff in the field. The main anxiety of those who oppose additional salary is that increment based upon training responsibilities mistakenly implies that students are more important than clients; disparity would add disadvantages to the additional burdens which may be imposed upon other staff, most of whom feel less favoured when they are not involved in training.

Support for the recognition of educational responsibilities in terms of salary but the need to see this in relation to the whole service came, from the Institute of Medical Social Workers.

> One essential factor in the development of field work placements is that salary scales should be structured in such a way that teaching commitments are recognised, and teaching qualifications adequately rewarded. . . . Payments alone however would only serve to increase the pressures on the supervisor. Unless teaching is part of the total plan for a department which is staffed appropriately for the work entailed, the result (i.e. of merely offering a higher salary) would be virtually to buy part of the supervisor's leisure time.

Events show recognition that the cost of supervision should not fall wholly upon the particular body offering training. There were differences of view about the just sharing of financial responsibility.

It was found that for student units (see Chapter 5, p. 85) the whole or a proportion of the cost of the salary of the supervisor might be met in certain services by the Treasury; and contribution to this cost may also be made when other members of the staff give considerable time to students not in units.

Some of the professional associations saw financial contribution as a means of encouraging training standards. The influence upon committees even of small grants was often mentioned and is underlined by several of the professional associations. The Association of Children's Officers write, after supporting the payment of adequate fees as a general principle:

> While so far the payment of fees in certain instances does not cover the staff time absorbed by the supervision of students, nevertheless some financial recognition for student training is valuable in persuading agencies to undertake a student training commitment particularly on a long-term basis.

A university lecturer with sixteen years of experience in a professional training course wrote:

> The recognition of student training services by special award . . . had beneficial effects, and one would like to see the practice extended to all the ministries concerned. It should encourage

more agencies to establish special supervisors' posts and to pay for them on grades at least commensurate with those for administrative responsibility.

Fees to voluntary agencies have been much discussed in recent years and a series of meetings was held during the period of the Survey under the auspices of the Standing Conference of Councils of Social Service.[1] The thirteen voluntary organizations providing practical work placements for students taking courses leading to the certificate in social work awarded by the Council for Training in Social Work have agreed to recommend a standard contribution reached by estimating the cost of weekly time given to students by members of the staff receiving a senior grade of salary. This decision was based partly upon the view that these organizations were supported by charitable funds given for purposes which do not include the training of students; it was, however, thought proper that voluntary agencies should offer their share of the cost by providing other amenities.

Accommodation

Sheer lack of physical space often prevents willing agencies and well qualified staff from offering supervision. The response of the whole staff towards students, and even teaching methods may be affected by rooms compulsorily shared, or in student units, by limits of space and comfort for other members of the staff. A number of the local authorities we visited had moved, or were about to be transferred from sometimes appallingly cramped quarters to new buildings, with much improvement for the regular staff. It was noticed, however, that even new city centres or shire halls had not always been designed so that individual interviews could take place in privacy, and sometimes when this provision had been made it was already threatened by increased staff. No doubt good training can be given under difficult physical circumstances, but the conditions under which the personal work of the staff is carried out must inevitably affect the attitude of clients, staff and students and the respect paid to important principles of confidence, undivided attention and courtesy.

In present students reports on 135 placements, about two thirds were sharing rooms with the staff, and in a third of these they thought the accommodation was poor. Their comments suggested great contrasts. Some conditions, putting it mildly, must discourage good work—

[1] The Standing Conference of Councils of Social Service, *Memorandum by the Working Party appointed by representatives of national voluntary casework organisations and representatives of Council of Social Service*, 1964.

for example: 'cubby hole'; 'no room—used various available corners'; 'squeezed in corner of big office and felt in the way'; 'one minute office for two of us, about 3 ft. 6 ins. wide'; 'sat at the desk of whoever was away; when the office was full, sat on the window sill'.

Two of the professional Associations thought that accommodation for students ought to be a justifiable claim upon central government training funds. This is not without precedent.

Clerical assistance

The shortage of qualified social workers lends special importance to secretarial help. The Survey showed astonishing variety in the amount of clerical time used by the staff in agencies where students were trained. Comparisons suggested that at least a fifth of the staff were spending precious hours which might have been saved if more clerical help had been provided. Wise use of time is essential for concentration on the heart of any social service, and students who have been encouraged to learn this during their training are likely to plan their work more economically when they are employed.

SUMMARY AND IMPLICATIONS

There are areas of the country where for no apparent reason few students are sent for field work. Concentration of students from basic courses in certain types of casework agency does not accord with the broader aims described by academic staff. Some social services of importance are only used for a negligible proportion of students from both types of course. There is increasing interest in community studies and group work though so far comparatively little development in these directions except for experience with groups in residential placements.

Considerable expansion might be brought about in settings and services not so far used. Advantages are likely to be gained for students from both professional and basic courses if some programmes are specially designed for each group. Staff appointments in the field for students undertaking community studies or placed in a variety of local agencies would help in expansion and in the coherence of their learning.

The full engagement of senior staff and committees in student training is seen as essential in spreading the range of responsibility and providing a balanced educational programme. More opportunities for study are needed for social workers in their own work and in relation to their students.

Financial recognition of training by subsidy from central public funds has been found essential to expansion of practical training in certain services. There is need also to include all field work in grants made to students, as well as for provision of adequate accommodation and clerical help.

7

LOOKING TOWARDS THE FUTURE

In this Survey certain facts about field work have been presented and an attempt made to reflect the main views of those concerned—the producers and the actors. Reviewers of a performance come to it with opinions about what is important to drama; their reviews might otherwise be as unprofitable as if they did not watch and listen receptively. There has, of course, been selection of situations and problems which seemed important in the experience of the authors, as well as in the theatres of social workers and those who train them. It has been possible only to indicate the more frequently expressed aims, difficulties and differences of view. Recording the main issues will, it is hoped, lead to further interest and debate, and clear the stage for further action.

In this chapter suggestions are made in the light of all the evidence, and the experience of those who carried out the survey.

It must first be repeated that the test of good education for social work lies in the further well-being of those for whom social services are designed. Preoccupation with training without continued study of how well these needs are or might be met recalls the definition of a fanatic as one who redoubles his efforts without reconsidering his aims. Further study of the nature and quality of social service is needed for appraisal of training.

There are signs of considerable changes of direction in the social services, calling for fresh thinking and enterprising action. Services hitherto concerned with specific needs or age groups are finding common cause in the wellbeing of the family;[1] social workers are being asked to draw upon all the resources of the community for individuals it is no longer content to 'put away';[2] closer relation

---

[1] Home Office, *The Child, The Family and The Young Offender*. H.M.S.O. Cmnd. 2742.
[2] See G. M. Carstairs, E. M. Goldberg, Margot Jefferys, Eileen Younghusband, R. Huws Jones, in *Care in the Community. The Fiction, the Reality and the Future*. Social Work, Vol. 22, Nos. 2 and 3, 1965.

is seen between the responsibilities of school teachers and social workers;[1] the prevention of delinquency relates to all these concerns. Effective training in the field is crucial in fitting students to meet these changes with imagination and competence.

The social worker must be able to see these developments from the standpoint of individuals and the relationships that most closely affect them; this has indeed been the main preoccupation of the staff in the types of field work reviewed. While individual understanding must remain at the heart of all social service, purposes may be defeated unless social workers also bring wisdom to bear upon social problems and social change. How, for example, are casework and other services to be made readily available to those who most need them, individually or in groups? What types of organization are effective for this purpose? How can citizens be enabled to find their own remedies? Can social workers from their intimate knowledge of human needs help in shaping social policy?

Education for social work is now the purpose of three national councils and a number of educational bodies, including universities, new and old, colleges of advanced technology, and local education authorities. The function of field work is actively discussed in a variety of patterns of training. What guidance follows from this study?

Evidence points all along the line to the need for clearer definition of purposes and more coherent planning of field work for students from basic courses. A considered sequence leading on to professional training, sufficient periods of time for different purposes in the field, and above all close relationship between practical work and study are essential to all types of course undertaken by those who intend to become social workers. Satisfactory relationship between study and practice means either that the same teacher must be able to turn from one to the other with understanding of both or that close partnership must be brought about between the staff responsible for field work and other studies. Field Study centres are provided for students of biology and kindred sciences. Why not for social studies? Might such centres, including staff experienced in social surveys, be a fruitful means of adding to the body of knowledge of social workers as well as to their discipline and skills and bringing into closer relation the study of social conditions, community development, group relations and family problems?

A considerable proportion of students who complete two years undergraduate certificates do not immediately proceed to professional training, and a number of those who enter social services never qualify.[1]

Could more incentive be given to these students to complete their training, by insistence as a condition of selection, or by changing the nature of the certificate so that it is clearly recognized as Part I of a training which can be completed only by taking a professional course, whether or not there is an intervening period of employment, marriage, or both?

The length and sequence of field work in courses for graduates in subjects other than social studies also calls for further consideration. This could be more coherently planned if the first year spent in the post-graduate diploma in social science followed by a second year in a professional course were designed as a whole. Useful evidence might be gained from a study of the experimental seventeen month courses offered by a few universities mainly for students entering the child care and probation services.

Events of the past five years have shown that courses in colleges of further education, in extramural university departments and other educational centres are meeting an urgent need for more trained staff. There is evidence that any considerable expansion in the number of trained social workers depends upon attracting men and women who do not hold qualifications for entry to the university as well as those who do. Some of the courses outside the university are designed particularly to attract older men and women, and some for staff who have been appointed as social workers without qualification and have had some years of experience. Different educational and practical problems in field training are set by mature men and women. Family responsibilities affect their availability for training and for employment. Experienced social workers approach training in a different way. Whatever allowance is made for experience, disinterested education and appraisal as well as the need for freshness of approach makes it essential for a period of field training to be undertaken in an agency other than the one in which they are employed.

These developments, which have gathered pace since the Survey was started, illustrate the varied and sometimes competing claims, calling for consideration of priorities.

Even if considerable expansion of opportunities for field training could be achieved by better distribution of students in terms of area and

[1] Barbara N. Rodgers, *The Careers of Social Studies Students*. The Codicote Press. Occasional Papers on Social Administration, No. 11, 1964. Tables II & III, pp. 12 & 13. Of the students who completed basic courses in 1960, 43 per cent had, by 1961 proceeded to professional training.

services, and by group teaching, casework services are likely to have more demands made upon them than they can meet. Three questions arise: What principles and standards should determine priorities? By what means could they be considered and kept under review by all the bodies concerned—national training councils, educational bodies, social agencies and professional organizations? What practical aids are needed and how could these best be provided?

It has already been suggested that there would be advantages if some agencies were to offer supervised experience suitable *either* for students from basic *or* from professional courses. There are no doubt good reasons in some services for different members of the same staff being concerned with students from one or other type of course; in some agencies however there seems much to be said for developing different programmes. In this way aims might be clearer, more suitable opportunities developed and communication between staff of courses and social workers made simpler and more effective.

Teaching units for those students who in any event undertake their field work at a distance from their courses might well be placed so as to develop training resources in relatively unused areas. It is not suggested that students from certain basic courses should be sent only to particular areas. There was strong feeling on the part of academic staff against any such boundaries, and with good reason. The intellectual and social development of young people may be enhanced either by gaining knowledge and confidence in familiar territory or by meeting the challenge of contrast. Choice ought not to be unnecessarily circumscribed.

Nevertheless, in the face of pressure in certain areas and services it seems essential that agency and staff fitted for professional education should give preference to students from professional courses. This implies agreement about standards; more knowledge about agencies prepared to give training, and more co-operation between those responsible for both types of course.

Even if the priority is accepted the future field work training of students from professional courses must depend to a considerable extent upon whether training for all social work will come to be regarded as indivisible or will continue to be provided in parallel courses, depending mainly upon practical training in and for particular services. If all casework services are used for all students different problems are presented in the logistics of placements and to some extent in methods of supervision.

The issue of generic and specific courses was a subject of discussion in many of our interviews. The methods of the Survey were not designed to provide an answer as to which method of training is the more effective. Differences of view are however in themselves important in planning for the future.

A number of Departmental and other reports have urged the need for more unified social service. From the point of view of long term economic planning for all the services of the country there is indeed a strong case for generic social work education. University courses in applied social studies are evidence of support for common professional training. Outside the universities experiments of a similar kind are taking place, as, for example, in a course where experienced health, welfare and child care officers train together, and their examination of specific needs and services is combined with the study and application of basic knowledge and principles. The report leading to the setting up of the Council for Training in Social Work and the National Institute for Social Work Training was concerned with local authority health and welfare services,[1] but they have attracted for consultation and common purposes representatives from all branches of social work and training. Professional associations increasingly recognize and discuss concerns they share.

In the Survey the staff responsible for generic courses and a number of social workers supervising their students were confident in the rightness of this approach. They were influenced, and convincingly so, by their own progressive discovery of facts, principles and methods essential to social work as they and their students shared study and experience. They saw also the merits of comparative experiences, and of flexibility in the choice of future employment by students not committed to a particular service.

The tutors of one course put the educational advantages emphatically in the following comment:—

> Nothing but advantage is seen in combined training of those who come from and go into varied agencies. Undoubtedly there are specialities and these have to be taught (e.g. delinquency and the importance of legal authority) but even here there are aspects of authority in different services (doctors in medical social work) and special skills are often not clearly distinguished or are really common to other services . . . students are found to be enriched immediately by their exchanges, and this heightens their interest in what they have in common. First they come as mental welfare

---

[1] Ministry of Health, *Report of the Working Party on Social Workers in Local Authority Health and Welfare Services.* H.M.S.O., 1959.

officers, child care officers, etc.; then they become social workers; then they become caseworkers, and finally they regard themselves as social workers again.

Some of the casework staff however expressed strong preference for receiving students who were proposing to enter their particular service. A few indeed felt strongly that the needs of any one service could be more effectively met if training courses tailored for this purpose were continued or even expanded.

There were arguments on both sides which related more to the practical needs of the social services than to principles and methods of education. Certain training bodies were driven by the urgency of providing quickly for their own services, even when they made full use of generic courses for some of their students. In this connection it was argued that recruitment is affected by the strength of incentives to enter a service designed to meet particular human needs such as those of deprived children, patients, or delinquents.

The keen sense of responsibility felt by staff for promoting and providing training for certain services, and their intimate knowledge of its needs and problems has positive value and should be respected in spite of the advantages of planning for social work as a whole. It may be that some students learn more effectively by focus upon particular services and others by the search for common knowledge and principles; this view is held by some experienced staff concerned with large numbers of students. It seems clear that both types of training—general and specific—will for the present continue; this diversity may attract more students and perhaps engage the help of social workers with varied interests and gifts. Incentives, however, change. A number of influences and the impressive experience of other countries, suggest that the change will be in the direction of more comprehensive services and training. Whatever these developments, it is of the utmost importance that extension of training for diverse services should be related to common aims and standards.

There are already precedents for agreement about priorities. Certain regional discussions between representatives of courses and agencies show readiness for a more rational approach in their common concern for training. Principal Probation Officers are encouraged to give certain preferences to students from approved university applied social studies courses, whether or not they intend to enter the probation service.

In view of the trend towards generic training the legal restriction on expenditure of public funds to training for specific services is anachronistic. It is, for example, a contradiction in terms that grants to students should commit them initially to employment in one service only, when they enter courses in applied studies, one of the purposes of which is to allow them freedom of choice. Ingenuity and goodwill in the transfer of responsibility for grant does not seem a sensible answer. There are other anomalies in financing training—for example, subsidies and fees to agencies—which emphasize the case for more unity and consistency between govenment departments supporting training.

In discussion of priorities the issue of concurrent and block training, considered in Chapter 6, is of obvious importance. Close and continuous association between the staff of courses and agencies has been shewn to have an essential bearing upon the spirit and methods of practical training. Developments important to staff and students are taking place as a result of this partnership, which it is difficult to create and maintain at a distance. There is therefore a strong case for giving priority in certain areas not only to professional courses as such, but also to those in which this partnership is valued and can be maintained. There are on other grounds practical and perhaps educational advantages in a variety of patterns provided they do not compete in a destructive way, and that effective consultation takes place between the staff of agencies and courses. For some time to come there will be a number of areas in which courses using concurrent field work are not established. These areas would provide a suitable choice for the establishment of units for students from professional courses placed for full time periods, or for special programmes for those sent from basic courses.

The rational consideration of these related needs and claims calls for consultation and co-ordination between organizations with diverse as well as common concern for the future of social services.

The three national training councils[1] were established by, or in relation to, statutes designed to provide qualified staff for particular services. Already the converging interests of these services and the contingencies of training have led to consultation and some mutual planning. It now becomes a matter of urgency from the standpoint of training in the field, to devise means by which common purposes could be furthered in the light of more unified social services, the need for comparable standards of training and the advantages of shared resources.

The universities have for many years had their own forum for dis-

---

[1] The Advisory Council for Probation and After Care and the Central Training Council in Child Care (Home Office); The Council for Training in Social Work.

cussion of common problems in departments of social study and administration, including field work, and it is here that consideration of the different claims on the social services of their basic and professional courses belongs. A channel of consultation is needed between the universities and other educational bodies concerned with training social workers; this is beginning to take place at the regional level.

Professional associations represent the interests both of the services and of training, and their evidence has shewn that they share many views about the ways in which standards of field work might be improved. Their 'Standing Conference'[1] is able to offer facts and views of importance to bodies promoting or carrying out training.

The staff of social agencies responsible for field work are indirectly represented in these organizations in a number of ways. The evidence of the Survey suggests however that senior staff responsible for public and voluntary services are at present not fully enough engaged in discussions of training policy and programmes.

Co-ordination at the national level and in consultation with educational bodies would, it is hoped, lead to more profitable use of public funds for the development of field work for all students of professional courses. In this Survey a number of suggestions for expansion have been made, involving special appointments for the teaching of groups of students and subsidies for certain educational purposes. These suggestions apply not only to local authorities, but to voluntary organizations. It has been seen, for example, that student units established in privately supported agencies have pioneered in the face of a precarious future, though security is essential for satisfactory development. Voluntary organizations were the creators of training for social work and it would be a serious loss to professional education if students were not able to experience the special nature of their service. Grants for their training programme would enable some agencies of good standard to make special teaching appointments and to provide for more students.

Discussions at national level could lead to recognition of certain standards for field work, such as those which are embodied in the memorandum sent to Children's Departments by the Central Training Council in Child Care.[2] In the United States the Department of Health, Education and Welfare, in consultation with the Council on Social

[1] Standing Conference of Organizations of Social Workers, 42 Bedford Square, London, W.C.1. See Annual Report, 1964.
[2] Central Training Council in Child Care, Home Office: *Memorandum of Guidance on the Practical Training of Child Care Officer Students* (unpublished), 1963.

Work Education, issues Guides for Field Instructions to agencies administering certain services, and distinguishes between the needs of students at different stages in their education for social work.[1] Such memoranda can provide valuable statements on principles and methods for discussion with agencies offering or being invited to undertake practical training.

Local co-ordination must also take place if field work resources are to be fully developed, and for this purpose it is essential that senior staff of the agencies be brought into consultation.

Common sense suggests that certain kinds of information should become available as a first step in finding out all the agencies able and willing to provide training. How could this information be assembled, kept up to date and made easily available to those who are making plans for students, so that it would aid and not interfere with direct relationship between the staff of courses and agencies?

One useful source of information is a register of the qualification and employment of their members maintained by professional organizations. There is at present only one association of social workers which publishes an annual list of this nature, and it appears to be fully used.[2] Professional qualification is not of course the only guide to competence for supervision but it is of primary importance to those who are placing students. Similar publication by all professional associations would be valued.

Another common sense approach would be to find out at regular intervals where students are placed in regions, and whether there are other services in which they would be welcomed. Certain counties and county boroughs already publish detailed accounts of their services. Might more information be assembled about opportunities for training? This knowledge and a great deal more is of course already available to certain national services through their local inspectorate, and to some professional organizations. Such communication is apt to run in parallel lines and may be considered in terms of a single area only when a new course is about to be established.

One suggestion worth experiment would be to set up in certain areas a small consultative group on field work, with an organizing secretary. This group might include individuals who represent services in the field, different types of training course, and the professional organizations. It would be necessary to establish the principle that they

[1] U.S. Department of Health, Education and Welfare. Anne Wilkens: *Guides for field instruction for graduate schools of social work, field experience of undergraduate students, and summer employment of undergraduate students*, 1963.

[2] The Association of Psychiatric Social Workers, 71, Albany Street, London, N.W.1.

I

were only to be concerned with the assembly of facts and not with the appraisal of services. Information important for training purposes could, however, be agreed centrally; for example, the number and qualifications of casework staff; their approximate work load; whether there was an in-service training programme; accommodation and clerical assistance. These records should be simple; easily brought up-to-date and classified.

There was evidence that many of the agencies would welcome the invitation to consider what type of training, if any, they could most usefully offer. Training Officers are being appointed by some local authorities to take responsibility for staff development and this will affect plans for students. Information about such appointments would be of value for all concerned with training.

A number of the academic staff members expressed doubt about the value of assembling what in the Survey enquiry were called 'formal facts' about agencies in which field work might be undertaken, either because they were placing students only with local agencies and knew enough about them, or because they thought that bare facts would be of little use without the personal exchange giving them life and meaning. Evidence showed, however, that when central information was available they were glad to make use of it.

In the chapter on expansion of training, reference was made to the need for further educational opportunities for the field work staff supervising students. Advanced courses are under discussion at some universities. They should fulfil an important need, particularly for staff responsible for student units and for training officers. For others the more flexible scheme of Training Fellowships for prospective tutors provided at the National Institute for Social Work Training serves a useful purpose. Initiated by grant from the Gulbenkian Foundation, they are also supported by the Home Office for child care tutors. They provide a six months' period of study and teaching practice, mainly for those who will become tutors in social work courses. There should be gains on both sides if it were possible for staff responsible for courses and for practical training to study together.

A number of suggestions have now been made for clearer definition of ends and means and for co-ordination. In social and educational developments there are always delicate balances to be achieved between freedom and mutual dependence. These balances call for finesse in a programme of training involving issues such as the urgent need for extended social service; academic freedom; professional principles, government policy.

In the field work training of today and as it is more likely to be tomorrow, lack of consultation seems bound to lead to pressures which will be more restrictive than certain limits to choice reached now, by agreement. Consultation is essential; the success with which it is undertaken will demonstrate the measure of common concern for the quality of all social service.

In the opening chapter reference was made to the use of the word 'professional' in the training of social workers. This Survey shows in social work a striving towards the more justifiable use of this term. It has been said that a professional person, in addition to his duty to submit himself to an approved standard of training and to a code of behaviour, must endeavour to integrate his own discoveries to the common body of knowledge. In the words of John Rickman, this means learning 'in due humility' from the older generation, giving 'without arrogance' to the next, and treating one's own generation 'with generosity, as equals'.[1]

The response to this inquiry of those who are teaching and learning showed eagerness for progress in this sense. Much careful thought is being given to educational responsibilities in social work. Nevertheless, certain risks to services and to professional standards can be seen and should be faced; risks that standard might too readily be sacrificed to number, or effective social service to the fascination of learning and using particular skills; that common aims might be frustrated by sectional rivalry, or skilled practice by academic aloofness.

Liveliness of interest and generosity of outlook encountered in this study give much hope for the future, but is not enough. Any claim to professional standard turns upon willingness to judge training in terms of its fitness to meet human needs; to recognize and constantly to add to knowledge essential to these needs; to make this knowledge available to practitioners and students and to offer social work education which will be the starting point for progressive learning, wisdom and skill.

SUMMARY OF FINDINGS AND SUGGESTIONS

I. *Co-ordination between organizations responsible for training*

1. Common purposes and problems call for regular consultation between national councils promoting the training of social workers, educational bodies providing courses and professional organizations.

2. The following main questions call for consideration:

[1] J. Rickman, 'Psychology in Medical Education, *British Medical Journal*, 6th September, 1947.

(a) The length and desirable standards for field training in courses leading to professional qualification.

(b) The extent to which priority should be given to the development of generic courses using a variety of field work placements.

(c) The geographical distribution of courses requiring concurrent field work.

(d) Methods of consulting with chief officers of public and voluntary social services about provision of field training.

(e) Means of assembling information about opportunities for field work in regions.

(f) Provision of opportunities for post-graduate study by qualified social workers. Fellowships and short courses for staff responsible for training in the field.

(g) Representations to government departments about the commitment of grant aided students to specific services and anomalies in subsidies to agencies and in meeting the costs of field work for students.

(h) Consideration of grants from public funds to enable voluntary organizations to expand with security their provision for students.

II. *Professional Courses*

3. Students from professional courses should have a prior claim upon social agencies able and willing to offer this standard of training.

4. In programmes of expansion, first consideration should be given to professional courses adopting concurrent field work.

5. The field work of students placed for block periods calls for more effective communication between the staff of courses and agencies, and for staff establishment which will enable this to be carried out.

6. Student units should be encouraged in agencies where conditions seem favourable both in public and voluntary services, if necessary aided by grants from national public funds.

7. In field training the teaching of casework should be more effectively related to the policy and administration of social services.

8. More students should gain experience of community care.

9. Encouragement should be given both to the in-service training of staff and to seminars provided for those who supervise students.

III. *Basic Courses*

10. University students of social studies who wish to become social

workers should be given more incentive to undertake professional training.

11. Supervisors of students coming from various types of basic course need clearer guidance from academic staff about the purpose of particular periods of field work.

12. Closer consultation is also needed between academic and field work staff about the experience that can be offered, about methods of supervision and about individual students.

13. Further opportunities for field work should be explored in areas to which relatively few students are sent.

14. Types of social work agency and other settings suitable for supervised experience could be further extended with the help of regional surveys.

15. Special appointments of field tutors in certain areas might enable a larger number of students to be supervised in a variety of social agencies.

16. Field study centres might provide, under skilled educational direction, for students studying social conditions as a background to social work training.

IV. *Social Work Agencies*

17. Senior officers of social services should be more closely identified with the development and methods of field training by consultation between them and the staff responsible for courses.

18. Programmes for the training of students need to be related to plans for staff development and continued learning in employment.

19. Social work staff supervising students should have their work load sufficiently reduced to enable them to give regular time to teaching and to attend staff meetings of courses.

20. The training programme of students should include the policy and administration of the service, and involve not only caseworkers, but other responsible staff.

21. Resources throughout the country could be more effectively used if information were assembled from agencies prepared to offer experience or training. A small regional consultative group with the assistance of an organizing secretary might serve this purpose. Appraisal would be the responsibility of training bodies.

22. Remedies should be sought for cramped accommodation and shortage of clerical help if these conditions hamper service to clients and the acceptance and training of students.

V. *Professional Associations*

23. Views about standards of field training shared by professional associations of social workers should be made available to organizations concerned with social work education.

24. The regular publication of the names and employment of qualified members would be useful in the expansion of training.

VI. *Research*

25. The need for research is evident throughout this survey. The relation between human needs and the services provided by social workers is basic to the study of their training. Courses of differing entry requirements, length and pattern call for studies of the selection of students, objectives, content, educational methods and subsequent achievement.

APPENDIX

METHODS OF THE SURVEY

General Methods

The study was approached in two main ways. One was to get evidence in certain areas about the practical work situation as a whole, both from the staff of courses and of social work agencies concerned with the training of students. The other was to consult in a more comprehensive way those responsible on the one hand for arranging the students' field work and on the other for providing it.

Two methods of inquiry were used—interview and correspondence.

Interviews were held with the staff of all courses and social agencies in two areas, a proportion of whom were concerned with the same students. This method was also used in a third area where there were no courses, and to which few students were sent. The staff of courses and of agencies where considerable numbers of students were trained were also interviewed.

Correspondence inquiries were used for all other purposes. These were sent to all courses in the United Kingdom and Eire; to agencies in seven counties receiving students at a distance from their courses, and to organizations of social workers and of the senior officers of certain services. An association of present students volunteered the results of their own questionnaire after consultation with the Survey staff.

Two types of correspondence inquiry were used. The first, sent to the staff of courses, was for assembling the facts about the placement of students in services and areas; the second, sent to courses, agencies and professional organizations, invited opinions about the main issues which had come to light during the interviews in Areas I and II.

These approaches and methods will now be described in more detail.

Field work placements

Facts about the placement of students in services and areas were essential as a basis and starting point for the whole Survey. It was therefore necessary to choose a precise period recently completed to represent a training year. The Survey was started in November 1963; the dates chosen were the twelve months beginning on 1 October, 1962 and ending on 30 September, 1963, referred to as the 'Survey year'. All the main figures relate to this period and it was these placements which determined the agencies consulted. The later correspondence inquiry called for some facts about subsequent developments.

In this inquiry a distinction was made between periods in the field of at least four weeks, and those that were shorter. This was partly in the interests of simplicity and partly because it was assumed that shorter placements must be mainly for observation.

Full particulars about these placements were received from 88 out of 89 courses (one of the 88 returns, owing to a delayed request, is not included in the figures).

Area studies

Areas I and II, situated in the south-west and in the north-east, were chosen because they included a variety of basic and professional courses and agencies receiving both local students and those sent from other parts of the country. The area boundaries were set by the distances to which students who undertook concurrent field work had travelled, but they also included the staff responsible for students of basic and professional courses sent from a distance.

Interviews in these areas were held in six counties and four county boroughs. These interviews allowed for the ventilation of problems which the staff thought should be considered in a survey of this kind and then covered a series of topics not tied to precise answers, such as the aims of training for students from various types of courses; the experience chosen and methods used; communications between the staff of courses and agencies; the advantages and disadvantages of groups of students and of concurrent and block placements. Senior staff of agencies were asked to complete in writing certain particulars, such as the qualifications of supervisors; the students for whom they had been responsible; the approximate time involved; accommodation and clerical help.

Number interviewed in Areas I and II

In these two areas interviews were held with the staff of ten courses in four different educational centres—universities (3); university extramural (1); colleges of further education (2); college of advanced technology (1). They comprised six professional and four basic courses. In the interviews with senior staff and other social workers, ten different types of agency were represented. In all, sixty-eight members of staff were seen in thirty-seven agencies. The services included were children's departments; family case work (voluntary); medical social work (hospitals and public health); national assistance; probation; psychiatric social work (mental hospital, child guidance clinic, public health); welfare departments. We did not see the staff of settlements or residential establishments, but within the boundaries set in Chapter I, all other social services were included if students had been undertaking practical work for at least four weeks.

Area studies were chosen partly because this enabled us to interview academic and field work staff concerned with the same students from local courses, most of whom undertook field work concurrently with study. Many of these agencies were also receiving students for full time periods from distant courses. There was advantage in this because it provided a basis of comparison for the staff of the agencies. It meant however that there was a more complete picture of both aspects of training in courses adopting the concurrent plan than there was of those in which students did full time field work. This we tried to remedy in other inquiries.

In Area III the net was cast more widely in order to discuss with the staff of agencies the possibilities of further training where few or no students had been received. The twenty public and voluntary agencies in which interviews were held included not only those listed for Areas I and II, but also in services concerned with education, employment, housing, industry and new town development. Interviews were also held with the staff of courses from which students had most recently been sent, all of which were outside the county.

These areas were chosen as illustrative of methods and problems in practical work and their inter-relationship. They were not 'samples' in any statistical sense and the interviews were not designed to provide a quantitative measure of the incidence of situations or opinions. Other approaches were necessary to discover whether the main issues had come to light and to get some indication of their importance. Three were adopted:

1. A second correspondence inquiry to all the courses in the country.

2. Interviews with the staff of courses and of agencies in which large numbers of students were trained, or in which student units were being provided.

3. A correspondence inquiry to the social agencies in certain

primarily rural areas to which students had necessarily been sent only from courses at some distance.

Inquiries to the staff of courses

Interviews. A total of twenty-two courses were represented by the staff interviewed in all these approaches: universities (10); colleges of further education in courses leading to the Certificate in Social Work (5); university extramural departments (3); other training bodies, such as the Probation Department and the Institute of Medical Social Workers (4).

Correspondence. The second correspondence inquiry to the staff of all basic and professional courses was returned by 59 out of 61 to whom it was sent. The difference between the figures given here and for the returns to the first inquiry is due to the fact that every type of course was differentiated in the first return even when it was sent from the same department, whereas in the second several courses were often grouped in one reply.

This second inquiry was designed to cover some issues common to the staff of basic and professional courses and some which differentiated between them. Both were asked, for example, to what extent their intake of students was affected by opportunities for field work; whether in the current year (following that of the Survey), students were being sent to agencies not used before; the methods by which they sought for and assessed the suitability of agencies; what difficulties were experienced. They were asked to give their views about means of progress in field work, such as special appointments for the supervision of groups of students; more centralized information about opportunities, and the provision for supervisors of more opportunities for study. Questions relating to the aims of field work and the communication between staff of courses and agencies were framed differently for basic and professional courses. This inquiry invited expressions of opinion supplementary to all questions or topics and many valuable comments were volunteered.

Staff responsible for new courses. The fact that the Survey was carried out at the National Institute for Social Work Training offered special opportunities for discussion with newly appointed tutors of courses in Colleges of Further Education who held Gulbenkian Fellowships. Their experience provided further evidence of methods and problems in finding suitable field work.

Inquiries to Social Agencies

Interviews. There were two main purposes in interviews held with the staff of agencies receiving a considerable number of students. One was that in these circumstances they were likely to hold considered views; the other, that for the purpose of expansion it was essential to study various ways in which students were grouped.

Most of these agencies were in the London area and, therefore, provided examples of certain conditions not characteristic of the areas in which other interviews had been held.

These interviews included senior staff and supervisors in area offices of two voluntary family casework agencies and one concerned with invalid children; three teaching hospitals and one child guidance clinic. A total of 99 interviews were held with the staff of social agencies in which students were supervised.

Correspondence inquiry

Areas I and II had provided a picture of the field work of students from a number of different courses, but because of the proximity of professional courses, most of the staff had in one way or another felt the influence of concurrent study and field work, even though they might not be receiving these students. This was also true of the agencies in the London area. It seemed likely that other facts and opinions might be found by consulting social workers in primarily rural areas, in which there were no courses and to which students could only go for full-time field work from a distance. For this purpose a correspondence inquiry was sent to all the thirty-four agencies to which students had been sent in seven counties.

These counties were widely scattered and included the north, south, east and west of the country. An attempt was made to find out whether they had more requests on behalf of students than they could accept; for which types of course they regarded the experience they could offer as most suitable; whether or not they preferred to have students already committed to their own service; what were their aims and methods in practical training and any difficulties they experienced. Certain particulars were asked about the qualifications of staff, caseload and accommodation. These included 44 area offices. Unfortunately, the returns to this inquiry were relatively incomplete: 22 out of 34 replies were received from the various agencies and 34 out of 44 from the total number of area offices. The relatively small proportion of returns may reflect a poorly designed or over-complicated inquiry; there was some evidence that it was based too closely upon issues discussed with agencies receiving larger numbers of students and, therefore, seemed inappropriate. Some wrote that pressure of time and not lack of interest accounted for their failure to reply. It seems likely that those who did respond were more concerned about training than those who did not.

Professional Organisations

Most members of professional organizations of social workers are concerned in one way or another with training. Many are supervising in the field; a number are teaching in courses; almost all have been students of social work. All the organizations are concerned with standards of training, though it is actually provided only by the Institute of Medical Social Workers. Members are attracted fresh from their training each year, and the associations are therefore in a position to draw upon recent experience of field work.

A correspondence inquiry was sent at a later stage to the nine professional organizations of social workers affiliated to the Standing Conference of Organizations of Social Workers.[1] This inquiry consisted of a number of statements of different points of view about certain issues which had so far seemed both important and controversial, and about which their opinions were invited. They were asked, for example, what they thought about the issue of 'slow motion' teaching on a few cases or of training more closely related to actual conditions of employment; the merits or demerits of training students in groups; the most effective means of communication with the staff of courses, and the extent to which senior administrative members of staff and committees should be involved in plans for practical training and its content. The associations were asked to distinguish the response of their members who had completed training as recently as 1962 or 1963. The assembly of replies was with one exception[2] left to the associations. Some canvassed members for individual opinions; others sent replies from committees concerned with training. Memoranda were received from seven organizations.

Organizations of Senior Officers

This inquiry was also addressed to three organizations of senior

[1] Association of Child Care Officers;* Association of Family Case Workers;* Association of Moral Welfare Workers;* Association of Psychiatric Social Workers;* Association of Social Workers; Institute of Medical Social Workers;* National Association of Probation Officers;* Society of Mental Welfare Officers; The County Welfare Officers' Society.* (*Memoranda received.)
[2] See Moon, Marjorie, *The First Two Years*, A Study of Work Experience of some Newly Qualified Medical Social Workers, The Institute of Medical Social Workers, 1965.

officers of the social services most involved in the training of social workers.[1] Some had carried out studies of such questions as the demand and supply of trained staff and had taken active part in many of the problems raised in this Survey.

Present Students

The initial plans did not include consultation with present students. To have judged the import of their views would have involved large numbers because of the variety of courses, field work placements and individual circumstances. We were grateful, however, for an offer to consult their members made by the Association of Social Work and Social Study Students, an organization with a membership at the time of 234 students in basic and professional courses at three universities and two colleges of further education in Scotland and the north of England. After discussion with the Survey staff, the students' committee designed and distributed their own questions, and much of the analysis of the ninety-four returns (45 per cent) was made by their secretary. Their inquiry was designed to find out how far students regarded their own field work as satisfactory. Their replies were mainly used to illustrate points of view about such matters as the choice of field work; opportunities for discussion with staff; the relation between study and practice, and reports on their work.

After this inquiry had been launched a more limited distribution of the same questions went to present students at another university, and a group of about a hundred students who had just returned to another college from their summer field work in 1964 were asked for their views on a few of the same issues.

Scotland, Ireland and Wales

All universities, colleges and other bodies responsible for courses for prospective social workers in the United Kingdom and in Eire received the same correspondence inquiries. It had from the outset been decided that interviews with the Survey staff could only be undertaken in England. It was therefore a valuable addition to the evidence when the Scottish Home and Health Department offered to carry out a similar study. Their interviews were held with a staff of nine of the eleven Scottish courses and with fifty-one supervisors of field work. Included in this survey were children's officers, medical and psychiatric social workers in a variety of settings; probation officers; social

[1] Association of Children's Officers;* Association of Directors of Welfare Services* Society of Medical Officers of Health. (*Memoranda received.)

workers in voluntary casework agencies and local authority health and welfare officers. The discussions followed the general scheme used for the Survey as a whole, but the Scottish staff made their own analysis and report. It was thought more satisfactory that the findings should be included in one publication though separate references are made to the Scottish findings in certain contexts.

Consultation was held with the Co-ordinating Committee for Social Work Training in Wales, and staff of Welsh courses were interviewed by the Survey staff, though it was unfortunately not possible to include the agencies responsible for field work.

Note on Method

The inquiry was designed to find out the main facts about the nature of field work, the distribution of students, the purposes, methods and difficulties of staff and suitable remedies for present problems. Limitations of time prevented the combination of this wide survey with a first hand study of the teaching content and methods of supervisors in the field, and the ways in which the progress of students was in fact assessed. Such studies, central to field training will it is hoped follow this preliminary inquiry.

The record of each interview was analysed to identify characteristic aims and methods, major agreements and differences of view; some of these findings could be further checked for consistency when in the written replies a three point scale was used to indicate the degree of importance attached to opinions. There were however, few clear cut issues in which it seemed possible or profitable to measure the extent of different points of view.

Reliance had to be placed mainly upon the internal coherence of the whole picture when all the varied sources of fact and opinion were brought together. It then appeared that certain issues, agreements and divergences of view tended to repeat themselves in a variety of contexts, and it is these that are presented against the background of the facts of field work.

Forms of Inquiry

Readers interested in more details of method can see the forms of inquiry at the Institute for Social Work Training, 5 Tavistock Place, London, W.C.1.

INDEX

PART I: GENERAL

PART II: ORGANISATIONS AND SERVICES

PART III: REFERENCES (Footnotes)

Page

Butler, Barbara, *The Two Months Placement for Social Studies Students*, Case Conference, Vol. 8, No. 2, 1961 28

Central Training Council in Child Care (Home Office), *Memorandum of Guidance on the Practical Training of Child Care Officer Students*, 1963 (unpublished) 128

Carstairs, G. M., *Care in the Community: New Tasks for Community Care in our Changing Society*, Social Work, Vol. 22, Nos. 2–3, 1965 121

Donnison, D. V., *The Teaching of Social Administration*, The British Journal of Sociology, Vol. XII, No. 3, 1961 27

Education, Ministry of, *Half Our Future*, A Report of the Central Advisory Council for Education (England), H.M.S.O., 1963 .... 18, 122

Goldberg, E. M., *Care in the Community: Working in the Community: What Kind of Help do People Need?* Social Work, Vol. 22, Nos. 2–3, 1965 121

Health, Ministry of, *Report of the Working Party on Social Workers in Local Authority Health and Welfare Service*, H.M.S.O., 1959 .... 12, 125

Home Office, *The Child, the Family and the Young Offender*, H.M.S.O., 1965, Cmd 2742 121

Home Office Probation Department, Tutor Officers' Bulletin No. 1, 1964 (unpublished) 82

Jahoda, Marie, *The Education of Technologists: an exploratory case study at Brunel College*, Tavistock Publications, 1963 11

Jeffreys, Margot, *Care in the Community: The Organization of Community Health and Welfare Services*, Social Work, Vol. 22, Nos. 2–3, 1965 121

Joint University Council of Social and Public Administration, *Education for Social Work in the Universities*, J.U.C. 16

Jones, R. Huws, *Care in the Community: The Fiction the Reality and the Future, Summary of the Conference*, Social Work, Vol. 22, Nos. 2–3, 1965 121

Jones, Kathleen, *A Review of University Social Studies Departments*, University of Manchester, 1963 (unpublished) 24

The Teaching of Social Studies in British Universities, Occasional Papers on Social Administration, No. 12, Codicote Press, 1964 15

Lloyd, A. K., *Field Work as Part of Undergraduate Preparation for Professional Education*, The Social Service Review, Chicago, Vol. XXX, No. 1, 1956 29

Moon, Marjorie, *The First Two Years*, A Study of the Work Experience of some Newly Qualified Medical Social Workers, The Institute of Medical Social Workers, 1965 140

Moscrop, Martha E., *In-Service Training for Social Agency Practice*, Toronto University Press, 1958 97

Rickman, John, *Psychology in Medical Education*, British Medical Journal, 6th September, 1947 131